PUBLIC HEALTH: PRACTICES, METHODS AND POLICIES

SCIENCE, CULTURE, AND POLITICS

DESPAIR AND HOPES IN THE TIME OF A PANDEMIC

PUBLIC HEALTH: PRACTICES, METHODS AND POLICIES

JOAV MERRICK - SERIES EDITOR

MEDICAL DIRECTOR, HEALTH SERVICES, DIVISION FOR INTELLECTUAL AND DEVELOPMENTAL DISABILITIES, MINISTRY OF SOCIAL AFFAIRS AND SOCIAL SERVICES, JERUSALEM, ISRAEL

Science, Culture, and Politics: Despair and Hopes in the Time of a Pandemic
Consolato M. Sergi (Editor)
2021. ISBN: 978-1-53619-816-4

Service Leadership Theory: Origin and Nature
Daniel TL Shek, Xiaoqin Zhu, Diya Dou and Joav Merrick (Editors)
2020. ISBN: 978-1-53619-389-3 (Hardcover)
2020 ISBN: 978-1-53619-430-2 (e-book)

The COVID-19 Pandemic: A Tribute to the Corona Whistleblowers
Joav Merrick, Søren Ventegodt and Niels Jørgen Andersen (Authors)
2020. ISBN: 978-1-53618-146-3 (Hardcover)
2020 ISBN: 978-1-53618-236-1 (e-book)

Public Health Themes in Grenada and the Caribbean Region
Joav Merrick and Lindonne Glasgow (Editors)
2020. ISBN: 978-1-53618-118-0 (Hardcover)
2020. ISBN. 978-1-53618-119-7 (e-book)

Advances in Chinese Children, Adolescent and Family Research
Ariel Tenenbaum, Daniel T.L. Shek, Moon YM Law and Joav Merrick (Editors)
2020. ISBN: 978-1-53617-870-8 (Hardcover)
2020. ISBN. 978-1-53617-871-5 (e-book)

Child Environmental Health Disparities: Looking at the Present and Facing the Future
I. Leslie Rubin and Joav Merrick (Editors)
2020. ISBN: 978-1-53617-823-4 (Hardcover)
2020. ISBN. 978-1-53617-824-1 (e-book)

Positive Youth Development: Digital Game-Based Learning
Ty Lee, Daniel T.L. Shek, Sarah Sw Lee, and Joav Merrick (Editors)
2020. ISBN: 978-1-53617-795-4 (Hardcover)
2020. ISBN. 978-1-53617-796-1 (e-book)

Service Leadership Education in an Era of Service Economy
Daniel TL Shek, Xiaoqin Zhu, and Joav Merrick (Editors)
2020. ISBN: 978-1-53617-514-1 (Hardcover)
2020. ISBN: 978-1-53617-515-8 (e-book)

Parenting and Family Life in a Chinese Society
Daniel TL Shek, Moon YM Law, Joav Merrick (Editors)
2020. ISBN: 978-1-53616-705-4 (Softcover)
2020. ISBN: 978-1-53616-706-1 (e-book)

Public Health: Topics, Themes and Trends
Satesh Bidaisee, Sadik Uddin Emmanuel Keku, Joav Merrick (Editors)
2020. ISBN: 978-1-53616-655-2 (Softcover)
2020. ISBN: 978-1-53616-656-9

Public Health: Environment and Child Health in a Changing World
I. Leslie Rubin and Joav Merrick (Editors)
2019. ISBN: 978-1-53615-394-1 (Hardcover)
2019. ISBN: 978-1-53615395-8 (e-book)

Service Leadership: Tools to Assess Knowledge, Attitude and Behavior
Daniel TL Shek, Xiaoqin Zhu, Li Lin and Joav Merrick (Editors)
2019. ISBN: 978-1-53614-852-7 (Hardcover)
2019. ISBN: 978-1-53614-853-4 (e-book)

Public Health Yearbook 2017
Joav Merrick (Editor)
2018. ISBN: 978-1-53613-792-7 (Hardcover)
2018. ISBN: 978-1-53613-793-4 (e-book)

Resilience and Health: A Potent Dynamic
I Leslie Rubin and Joav Merrick (Editors)
2018. ISBN: 978-1-53613-412-4 (Hardcover)
2018. ISBN: 978-1-53613-413-1 (e-book)

Medical History: Some Perspectives Second Edition
Donald E. Greydanus and Joav Merrick, (Editors)
2018. ISBN: 978-1-53613-319-6 (Hardcover)
2018. ISBN: 978-1-53613-320-2 (e-book)

University Students: Promotion of Holistic Development in Hong Kong
Daniel TL Shek, Lu Yu and Joav Merrick (Editors)
2017. ISBN: 978-1-53612-535-1 (Hardcover)
2017. ISBN: 978-1-53612-537-5 (e-book)

Alzheimer's Disease: Awareness among Young Adults
Ronald Chow, Drew Hollenberg, Michael Borean and Joav Merrick (Editors)
2017. ISBN: 978-1-53612-456-9 (Softcover)
2017. ISBN: 978-1-53612-457-6 (e-book)

Service Leadership Education for University Students
Daniel TL Shek, Po Chung, Li Lin and Joav Merrick (Editors)
2017. ISBN: 978-1-53611-949-7 (Hardcover)
2017. ISBN: 978-1-53611-969-5 (e-book)

Leadership: Promoting Leadership and Intrapersonal Development in University Students
Daniel TL Shek, Cecilia MS Ma and Joav Merrick (Editors)
2017. ISBN: 978-1-53611-950-3 (Hardcover)
2017. ISBN: 978-1-53611-970-1 (e-book)

Caribbean Adolescents: Misuse and Abuse of Alcohol
Cecilia Hegamin-Younger and Joav Merrick (Editors)
2017. ISBN: 978-1-63485-880-9 (Hardcover)
2016. ISBN: 978-1-63485-894-6 (e-book)

Public Health: An Ecological Framework for Child Environmental Health Interventions
I. Leslie Rubin and Joav Merrick (Editors)
2017. ISBN: 978-1-53610-700-5 (Hardcover)
2017. ISBN: 978-1-53610-714-2 (e-book)

Diabetes Mellitus: A Medical History Journey
Donald E. Greydanus and Joav Merrick
2016. ISBN: 978-1-53610-094-5 (Softcover)
2016. ISBN: 978-1-53610-103-4 (e-book)

Education in Hong Kong: Service Leadership for University Students
Daniel TL Shek, Cecilia MS Ma, Li Lin and Joav Merrick (Editors)
2016. ISBN: 978-1-63484-928-9 (Hardcover)
2016. ISBN: 978-1-63484-960-9 (e-book)

Environmental Health Disparities: Costs and Benefits of Breaking the Cycle
I. Leslie Rubin and Joav Merrick (Editors)
2016. ISBN: 978-1-63484-211-2 (Hardcover)
2016. ISBN: 978-1-63484-212-9 (e-book)

Higher Education in Hong Kong: Nurturing Students to be Caring Service Leaders
Daniel TL Shek, Andrew MH Siu, Hildie Leung and Joav Merrick (Editors)
2016. ISBN: 978-1-63484-980-7 (Hardcover)
2016. ISBN: 978-1-63485-009-4 (e-book)

Measles: Epidemiology and Control of Measles in the Gweru Urban District in Zimbabwe
Tawanda Marufu, Seter Siziya, Mazyanga L. Mazaba and Joav Merrick (Editors)
2016. ISBN: 978-1-63485-559-4 (Hardcover)
2016. ISBN: 978-1-63485-573-0 (e-book)

Medical History: Some Perspectives
Donald E. Greydanus and Joav Merrick
2016. ISBN: 978-1-63484-747-6 (Hardcover)
2016. ISBN: 978-1-63484-849-7 (e-book)

Public Health: Some International Aspects
Joav Merrick (Editor)
2016. ISBN: 978-1-63484-612-7 (Hardcover)
2016. ISBN: 978-1-63484-630-1 (e-book)

Public Health: International Aspects on Environment and Health
I. Leslie Rubin and Joav Merrick (Editors)
2016. ISBN: 978-1-63484-834-3 (Hardcover)
2016. ISBN: 978-1-63484-849-7 (e-book)

Smoking and Adolescence: International Public Health Experiences
Mazyanga L. Mazaba, Seter Siziya and Joav Merrick (Editors)
2016. ISBN: 978-1-63484-311-9 (Hardcover)
2016. ISBN: 978-1-63484-312-6 (e-book)

Arbovirus: Public Health Experience from Zambia
Seter Siziya, Mazyanga L. Mazaba, and Joav Merrick (Editors)
2015. ISBN: 978-1-63463-601-8 (Hardcover)
2015. ISBN: 978-1-63463-618-6 (e-book)

Health Issues in Diverse Cultures
Cecilia Obeng, Samuel Gyasi Obeng and Joav Merrick (Editors)
2015. ISBN: 978-1-63463-613-1 (Hardcover)
2015. ISBN: 978-1-63463-619-3 (e-book)

Public Health, Social Work and Health Inequalities
Bruce D. Friedman and Joav Merrick (Editors)
2015. ISBN: 978-1-63482-838-3 (Hardcover)
2015. ISBN: 978-1-63482-850-5 (e-book)

Patient Dumping: Background, Protections, and the Mentally Ill
Tabitha E. Rivers (Editor)
2015. ISBN: 978-1-63483-726-2 (Hardcover)
2015. ISBN: 978-1-63483-727-9 (e-book)

Tomorrow's Leaders: Service Leadership and Holistic Development in Chinese University Students
Daniel TL Shek, Andrew MH Siu and Joav Merrick (Editors)
2015. ISBN: 978-1-63321-880-2 (Hardcover)
2014. ISBN: 978-1-63321-943-4 (e-book)

Environment and Public Health: Environmental Health, Law and International Perspectives
I. Leslie Rubin and Joav Merrick (Editors)
2014. ISBN: 978-1-63463-167-9 (Hardcover)
2014. ISBN: 978-1-63463-189-1 (e-book)

PUBLIC HEALTH: PRACTICES, METHODS AND POLICIES

SCIENCE, CULTURE, AND POLITICS

DESPAIR AND HOPES IN THE TIME OF A PANDEMIC

CONSOLATO M. SERGI

nova science publishers
New York

NOTICE TO THE READER

Library of Congress Cataloging-in-Publication Data

ISBN: 978-1-53619-816-4

Published by Nova Science Publishers, Inc. † New York

To our children and youth, because respect for traditional values, education, and tolerance will be key to make them "stronger together."

CONTENTS

PREFACE

In June 2021, new waves and variants of the current COVID-19 pandemic are still messing up our lives and magnetizing the compass of our existence. No other epidemics or pandemics have been politicized at such a level since ancient times. The political spectrum from right to left has tried to ride this pandemic and upset the public health response efforts. Statistics and politics have changed our daily approach to this infection. Cruel has been the palpable miscommunication. Massive and uncontrolled lockdowns have jeopardized the economy of our planet. In this book, the author analyzes the pandemic in a historical context, emphasizes the importance of facemasks, but also highlights the substrates of an anti-mask psychology. It would be appalling to call mistakes in public health decisions "learned lessons" because it reduces the gravity of the consequences of inadequate communication. Our youth is our future. The mental issues arising from a lack of social interaction and in-person education are dreadful. Vaccines are powerful and represent the most outstanding progress in medicine. However, intolerance against vaccine opponents and hesitant families has been vocalized with martial tones in both social media and news channels raising doubts on true freedom of speech. There is, indeed, light at the end of the tunnel, but vaccine acceptance or herd immunity is not the answer, or probably, not the only one. There is some evidence that we are going back to our ancient world with iconoclastic tones. The COVID-19 pandemic may be an occasion to reconsider the traditional family and values in the center of our lives and daily politics. A tolerance towards any race needs to be contagious, militant, and blazing to rebuild and revitalize the American Dream vehemently.

INTRODUCTION

At the end of the fourth century, a unique collection of letters circulated in Europe. It occurred some time after the Milan edict of the proclamation of religious tolerance for Christianity within the Roman Empire of 313 AD. The epistolary collection was composed of eight letters from the philosopher Seneca to the apostle Paul and six letters of response from the apostle to his correspondent. Remarkably, not only was the collection believed to be authentic, but it received good support from thinkers and academicians, such as Jerome [1]. Seneca seems to consider himself already Christian and emphasizes the cure of the style in his epistolary intercourse with the Apostle. Now, this collection is deemed fake. However, this correspondence may suggest the fortune that Seneca's moral philosophy encountered in Christian environments. It constitutes an invitation for non-Christian people to ponder on the apostle's letters. Notably, it attempted to seek some point of mediation between classicism's rhetorical education and the ascendant religion's literary devotion. This fake correspondence may also reveal how crucial it was to gain support for the new religion from academicians at that time. The mutual understanding of the two cultures was challenging. The new faith was raising communicability issues that will resonate for many centuries ahead. In the 4th century, Julian was the last non-Christian ruler of the Roman Empire, believing that restoring the Empire's ancient Roman values and traditions was necessary to save it from dissolution. It was a turbulent time. Cultural and spiritual processes lead, eventually, Christianity to incorporate some attitudes and values of the pagan world. Still, the search and necessity of bridges were evident, and the fake correspondence may have been one of these attempts. The authenticity of the correspondence between the philosopher Seneca and Paul was debated for several centuries. These letters started to be considered falsified in the 15th century. Historiography documents that the chronological errors, visible poverty of thought and style, and the conception of the relative positions of the Stoic School and the rising Christian religion should deceive the forger [2].

I started this book by mentioning the event of this classical historical apocryphal text because it may representone of the early "fake news" of our Western heritage. It is also important to emphasize that such connotation does not decrease the influence of any faith. It is part of our nature to create bridges. Still, it underlines that good thoughts and perceptions may quickly invalidate some lines of thought. Also, it reminds us that veridicality and authenticity of any document need a careful and conscientious process to avoid that allegations remain unfounded diffusing doubts on institutions or people. Between 1887 and 1917, Sherlock Holmes appears in Sir Arthur C. Doyle's novels. The real-life figure of Joseph Bell, a Scottish general surgeon working actively at the Royal Infirmary of Edinburgh, inspired these stories. Sir Doyle met him in 1877 and worked for him as a clerk. Holmes' figure carries a distinct position in Western literature as one of detective fiction's most influential texts. It reminds us to separate data from interpretation carefully. Sir Doyle learned this when working at the Scottish hospital. Sherlock Holmes' techniques focused on footprints, decryption of symbols, and meticulous analysis of handwriting. Holmes was clearly at the vanguard of innovation in solving crimes using several methods. In our society, it seems that we often jump to conclusions raised by perceptions. Such an approach leaves us to interpretative decisions that may undermine the absolute authenticity of texts and events [3]. During the current pandemic, some public health officials, politicians, and academicians have shown a sprezzatura, which is terrifying.

Massimo Troisi was an Italian actor who passed away at 41 years, a few days before the scheduled cardiac surgery following a rheumatic fever that damaged his heart when he was a child. Massimo Troisi had one of the best friends in Roberto Benigni, who directed "*Life is Beautiful.*" Massimo Troisi was born in San Giorgio a Cremano, in the Neapolitan province of Italy. He was shy, controlled, and often spoke softly. The heart attack that destroyed the actor's life occurred after shooting his most important and "international" movie, *Il Postino* (The Postman). His death has given this actor and his film to the legend before even being released in theaters. Troisi received two *postmortem* Oscar nominations for Best Actor and Best Non-Original Screenplay. Troisi introduced Italy to the world in a Neapolitan spirit devoid of pizza, spaghetti, and mandolins. His humor was full of dramatic excesses, often whispered and devoid of clichés. The transition from the lounge to movie theaters started in 1981 with "*Ricomincio da Tre.*" Massimo immediately conquered audiences and critics, as well as two David of Donatello (best film and best actor) and two Silver Ribbons (best subject and best new director). In this movie, Troisi recounts the Neapolitan boy Gaetano (Troisi), who, tired of his ordinary life, decides to move to Florence. Here, he will meet Marta, to whom he is immediately attracted. This movie, which condenses situations more than a linear story, discloses sentences, which will stay in the memory for generations. Troisi deals with various topics in the movie, including friendship, love, jealousy, betrayal, mental illness, family relationship, discomfort in a raging and individualistic society [4].

The dialogues of the protagonist with his friend, Lello, remain universal.

Gaetano: That is, if I'm telling you that I'm leaving, I'm leaving ... and then I go Rafè, I can't anymore! That is, what has been, has been, enough! So I start again from three! (*Cioè, se ti sto dicendo che parto, parto... e poi me ne vaco Rafè, nu ci'a faccio cchiù! Cioè, chello che è stato, è stato, basta! Ricomincio da Tre!*)

Lello: From scratch! (*Da zero!*)

Gaetano: *Eh?*

Lello: From scratch! Do you start from scratch? (*Da zero! Ricominci da zero!*)

Gaetano: No please, I start again from three, because three things I know I managed in my life. Why do I need to lose them too?! Shall I restart from scratch?! From three! ... I go to restart again, I can't anymore... (*Nossignore, ricomincio da... cioè, tre cose me so' riuscite ind'a vita, pecchè aggià perdere pure cheste?! Aggià ricominciare da zero?! Da tre!... Me ne vaco, nun ci'a faccio cchiù...*).

The concept is fundamental because we do not restart from scratch most of the time, but from things that have been important in our lives and kept in our hearts and souls wherever we go. The current pandemic is also a way to reflect on these aspects, despair, and hopes. We have the opportunity to think about ourselves, introspect our souls, and restart again. What is durable and unique that we would like to keep will be crucial for our re-growth. Two of these are love and solidarity. This book is more a quest for humanity. Being equanimous, sober, and calm in distress is very challenging. Not claiming the impossible with the heart is exceptionally arduous because the irrational cry in a flamboyant stage desire is almost always louder than the rational [5]. The morality in science, culture, and politics does not differ. It consists of the resistance to be seduced by allegorical or baroque words. In simplicity, the nonessential and noisy fragments are stripped away, and the individual focuses energy on events and things that matter the most.

Chapter 1

Epidemics and Pandemics

Abstract

This chapter presents a short history of epidemics and pandemics in a historical setting with some original texts and how people reacted to death over the centuries. The original text from Boccaccio's Decameron, a history of the pandemics, the most updated knowledge on the current severe acute respiratory syndrome – Coronavirus 2 (SARS-CoV-2) pandemics, and the role of inflammation in Coronavirus Disease 2019 (COVID-19) are elucidated.

Keywords: severe acute respiratory syndrome – Coronavirus 2, SARS-CoV-2, Coronavirus disease 2019, COVID-19, black death, plague, pandemic

To the great multitude of bodies shown, which to each church every day and almost every hour, not the sacred earth is sufficient for burials. Since we want to give each place its own sacrality according to the ancient custom and considering that the cemeteries of the churches were full, very large holes were digged in which hundreds of bodies were stowed in the guise of merchandise stuffed in ships, with some land on the top [*Alla gran moltitudine de' corpi mostrata, che a ogni chiesa ogni di e quasi ogn' ora concorreva portata, non bastando la terra sacra alle sepolture, e massimamente volendo dare a ciascun luogo proprio secondo l' antico costume, si facevano per gli cimiterii delle chiese, poi che ogni parte era piena, fosse grandissime nelle quali a centinaia si mettevano i sopravegnenti: e in quelle stivati, come si mettono le mercatantie nelle navi a suolo, con poca terra si ricoprieno infino a tanto che la fossa al sommo si pervenia*] [6-9]. This lugubrious text is from the Decameron of the 14th-century Italian writer Giovanni Boccaccio. The text subtitled *Prince Galehaut* (*Prencipe Galeotto*) was considered set against Dante Alighieri's "Divine" Comedy and labeled the "Human Comedy." The Decameron comprises 100 tales during societies, events, and passions, particularly tumultuous in the 14th century. The narratives are told during a self-inflicted lockdown by seven young women and three young men in an isolated villa just outside Florence when the Black Death devastated the city. The Decameron is probably conceived after the Northern Italy plague epidemic of 1348 and concluded by 1353 [10]. In the literary mosaic, tragic stories are admixed to erotic novellas with wit, jokes, and life lessons accents. This book provides a curious snapshot of life in the late Medieval period. Remarkably, the medieval narratives present in the Decameron show congruences and incongruences, probably not entirely dissimilar from some speculations, science, pseudoscience,and conspiracy theories driving the current pandemic.

Epidemiologically, an epidemic is a disease that involves a large number of individuals within a community, region, or general population. Conversely, a pandemic is an epidemic, which has been disseminated over multiple countries or continents [11]. The Gram-negative *Yersinia pestis* is the bacterium responsible for the deadly zoonotic disease. The plague has devastated societies for at least 5,000 years with intermittently more or less stable foci in the Americas, Africa, Europe, and Asia [12]. Historically, *Y. pestis* genomes have been recovered from affected archaeological sites, confirming multiple societies' burdens along the centuries. It has been suggested that such findings point out a progressive clonal evolution from a common ancestor. In history, three plague pandemics have been described. They include the Justinianic plague (541–750 AD), the Black Death, which began in the 1340s, and the third pandemic, which spread worldwide from

China at the end of the 18th century [12, 13]. The third plague pandemic has become primarily dormant, with hundreds of people being reported predominantly in some impoverished African countries [12, 14, 15]. This disease is called zoonotic because it is an infectious disease caused by a microorganism that has jumped from an animal to a human. The term zoonosis derives etymologically from Greek (ζῷον "animal" and νόσος "disease"). In the United States and Canada, zoonoses of most apprehension comprise brucellosis, Lyme disease, rabies, salmonellosis, West Nile virus infection, and the emerging coronavirus infections. These last infections include the Middle East respiratory syndrome or MERS and severe acute respiratory syndromes 1 and 2 (SARS-1 and SARS-2). Some of these zoonoses are urbanized, while others are primarily centered in rural regions. Substantially, six out of every ten infectious diseases in people seem to be zoonotic [16]. In a growingly interconnected world, it has been suggested to implement the medical and societal response to these zoonoses using a "One Health" approach [17]. "One Health" is a tactic that recognizes the connection between people, animals, plants, and their shared environment. This approach calls for experts in human, animal, and environmental health to work together to achieve the best health outcomes for everybody.

Plague is mainly transmitted to people by rodent-associated flea bites. The Justinian Plague, regarded as the first deadly pandemic, ravaged the Mediterranean Basin from 541 to 750/767 AD [12, 15]. It overran northern Europe. The "Black Death" pandemic is the second community infection of *Y. pestis* spanning 1346 to 1353. It has been approximately estimated that this second pandemic killed about one-third of the European population. Although primarily concentrated in the seven years of the 14th century, some data indicate that it persisted at least inconsistently for a few more centuries. The Chinese province of Yunnan was probably at the origin of the third plague pandemic, which began in 1772. The third plague spread worldwide on the eve of the 20th century following human movement via steamships and railroads. The *Y. pestis* microorganism was scrupulously discovered in Hong Kong in 1894 by the Swiss-French physician Alexandre Yersin, affiliated with the Pasteur Institute. The Institut Pasteur is a non-profit, privately funded international center in Paris, France. It stands out for investigations in biology, microbiology, and immunology. Remarkably, Dr. Yersin also contributed to resolving part of the cycle of transmission of this bacterium involving the rat (*Rattus rattus*) and its ectoparasite (*Xenopsylla cheopis*) [12, 15, 18, 19].

Infected flea bites are the main transmission, which occurs from one host to another and induces typically enlarged, warm, and painful lymph nodes underneath some reddened skin areas. These aspects of the affected lymph nodes remind the *tumor* (swelling), *rubor* (redness), *calor* (heat), and *dolor* (pain) features of inflammation. To these signs, which were initially recorded by the Roman encyclopedist Celsus in the 1st century AD, the *functio laesa* or loss of function was subsequently added. The affected lymph nodes are commonly referred to as *buboes* (Greek: βουβών, 'groin'), which is lymphadenitis or acute inflammation of the lymph nodes [20]. Bubo is an example of reactive lymphadenopathy. Lymphadenitis is followed by septicemic dissemination of the microorganism. At its portal of entry, *Y. pestis* may cause skin ulceration, reported as carbuncles and ulcers, along with bumps, petechiae, bruising, and gangrene [21]. The droplet inhalation after close contact with infected mammals generates the *primary pneumonic plague*. Similarly, the consumption of contaminated raw meat may cause *pharyngeal* and *gastrointestinal* plague. The outbreak control consists of point-of-care diagnosis, early antibiotic treatment, and confinement measures, the so-called "lockdowns" [22-24]. In a nutshell, the five principal forms of plague are bubonic, pneumonic, meningeal, pharyngeal, and septicemic. Different routes of interhuman transmission and human infection from plague sources have been precisely evidenced. They include nonhuman flea bites, transcutaneous contamination by carcass skinning, aerosol transmission, and raw or poorly cooked meat consumption. These routes of communication and the surrounding events have been immortalized in books and movies. Transmission occurs through aerosols and ectoparasites. Examples are the body and head lice and human fleas (*Pediculus humanus corporis* and *Pulex irritans*) [12]. The transmission via droplet was probably the pattern observed during the Manchurian plague outbreak of 1910 to 1911. The 1924-1925 Los Angeles plague outbreak is thought to have been pneumonic. It was highly contagious, but quarantine measures were not particularly effective [12, 15, 19].

Dr. Yersin's impact has been paramount in microbiology and immunology. It is important to recall his contribution to humanity. Dr. Yersin became the first physician to develop an antiserum to treat patients affected by the plague. He extensively collaborated with Drs. Calmette, Roux, and Borrel at the Pasteur Institute in Paris [12, 15, 19]. In 1896, Dr. Yersin treated 23 Chinese patients affected by the epidemic, and only two of these patients died. These encouraging data led other physicians to opt for this treatment. Caveats were, however, the lack of standardization among the methods they applied with a vast diversity of the outcome. The animals used for antiserum production and the variation in the doses given were not fully standardized according to Good Laboratory Practice (GLP) [15]. These limitations with some unsuccessful treatments led to unconvincing results and skepticism, which fostered some conspiracy theories. Nevertheless, antiserum continued over a decade in Africa, Asia, and South America. Eventually, it was credited a success. Dr. Yersin's contribution probably reduced mortality from 82% without treatment to 32% following the application of the antiserum. In Egypt, just a year after World War II (WWII), the antiserum was coupled with *sulfapyridine*. The combination resulted in only 12 of 69 plague patients who succumbed. Later, other drugs proved to be excellent over the antiserum. *Streptomycin* was used in India and Argentina. In the early 1950s, *chloramphenicol* and *oxytetracycline* were used, showing the same efficiency as *streptomycin*. Nephro- and ototoxicity limited the use of *streptomycin*, despite its still current use in Madagascar. *Gentamicin*, another aminoglycoside alone or in combination with *tetracycline,* was an acceptable substitute. According to World Health Organization (WHO) and the United States Center for Disease Control and Prevention (CDC) recommendations, antibiotics that are commonly used against *Enterobacteriaceae* are also demonstrated to be profoundly effective against plague if given promptly. Antibiotic therapy shows a clinical improvement within 2-3 days and needs to be continued for up to two weeks. In the case of septicemic plague, supportive treatment should be undertaken to limit the damage of vital organs.

Historians have struggled to find pandemics of the ancient periods apart from the above well-documented epidemical narratives. It remains challenging to recognize the clinical symptoms of plague by reading rare and imprecise available sources [12]. The descriptions of Greek and Chinese authors are vivid but still uncertain. Also, some sources may report epidemics originating from an entirely different microorganism lacking any current microbiological confirmation. It seems that the most ancient record of a plague outbreak is in the Old Testament in the Book of Samuel, where the plague was interpreted as a Divine punishment. In this text, the disease extended to Philistines in retaliation for the theft of the Ark of Covenant. Apollo was one of the Olympian deities in early Greek and Roman religions. Homer, the ancient author of the *Iliad* and *Odyssey*, describes an outbreak of plague driven by Apollo against the Greek army of Agamemnon, the king of Mycenae. When Helen was taken to Troy by Paris, Agamemnon commanded the united Greek armed forces in the Trojan War. Chryses, Apollo's priest, comes to the Greek camp to release his daughter, Chryseis, held captive by Agamemnon. Agamemnon insulted and sent Cryseis away, and Apollo sent a plague on the Greeks. Sophocles described the Plague of Thebes in the tragedy *Oedipus Rex*. It seems to be attributable to an infection due to *Brucella abortus*. This gram-negative microorganism causes brucellosis, a zoonosis mainly due to ingestion of undercooked meat or unpasteurized milk from infected animals. According to some documents, the Plague of Athens reported by Thucydides in 430 to 426 BC may have been typhoid fever. The Plague of Syracuse was an outbreak chronicled in 396 BC. Here, the infection decimated the Carthaginian army during the siege of the city. Diodorus Siculus reported that "*the plague first attacked the Libyans, and, as many of them perished, at first they buried the dead, but later, both because of the multitude of corpses and because those who tended the sick were seized by the plague, no one dared approach the suffering*" [25]. The sinister images include the stench of the unburied and the diffusion of the miasma theory. In depicting the Syracusan plague, Diodorus demonstrates a similarity of the symptoms endured by the Greeks during the Plague of Athens. The individuals exhibit swelling in the throat with catarrh production and burning painful sensations in the back with pustules upon the whole surface of the body. The Antonine Plague of the 2nd century killed approximately 10% of the Roman population and may have played a substantial role in initiating the decline of the Roman Empire. Galen witnessed this outbreak, but critical reading of his texts may favor smallpox as a probable etiological agent. Smallpox was an infectious disease due to a virus of the *Poxviridae* family. Later, the Plague of Cyprian, named after the bishop of Carthage, took place on the periphery of the Mediterranean sea between 249 and 262 AD. It has been speculated that the agent of this plague may have been smallpox, Ebola virus, or influenza [26, 27].

Marcus Tullius Cicero was a Roman statesman, writer, scholar, and lawyer who played an essential role in the politics of the late Roman Republic. Paraphrasing him in *De Oratore*, history may be personified as a teacher [28, 29]. We can better behave in the current time by reading history and avoiding committing past mistakes (*Historia magistra vitae est*). In reviewing the history of pandemics, I came across to the notion that both humans and infectious diseases have spread across the world and our missteps have been carried on with us [30]. The increase of the rural communities may have played a role in scaling up the number of epidemics and pandemics. The widespread trade created new chances for humans and animals to interact, speeding up the diffusion of these infections. The larger the urbanization becomes, the more exotic the business is, and the increase of routes has favored several potential areas where zoonoses can occur. Epidemics and pandemics throughout history increased, but there has been a gradual reduction in the death rate. It is critical to improve healthcare, introduce antibiotics, and implement safe trade and quarantine restrictions for boats and ships to sit at anchor before landing, as identified in mathematical models [31]. Still, a desire for humanity needs to pervade humans. In ancient times, spirits and gods have been considered inflicting or favoring disease and destruction upon those that deserved their wrath. This perception can be identified in Greek, Roman, and Medieval texts, but it has been present also in the most recent epidemics and pandemics. In Justinian's plague, the Byzantine historian Procopius of Caesarea tracked the plague's origin to East Asia. The historian acknowledged geography and trade's role in this spread but accused the Emperor Justinian. He proclaimed him to be either a devil or an individual who attracted God's punishment for his evil acts. The Justinian plague has been considered a trigger event, which thwarted the imperial efforts to reunite the Western and Eastern remnants of the Roman Empire.

Public health experts often use R0 (R naught) to mandates rules for public safety. This parameter is a fundamental measure to track the infectiousness of a disease called the "reproduction" number, which indicates how many susceptible individuals, on average, each sick person will, in turn, infect [32-34]. One of the most contagious diseases is measles harboring an astonishing R0 in the range of 12-18. In simple words, an individual can infect, on average, 12 to 18 people in an unvaccinated setting population. Measles is considered most virulent, but vaccination efforts and herd immunity can limit its spread. Vaccinations are critical because they prevent the virus from increasing, and the resurgence of known and treatable diseases becomes a mirage. Changing from nomadic life and small hunting to rural and then urban gathering with multimillion metropolises has been radical for the human being. Humanity relies on interindividual collaboration to avoid initiate and spread diseases that can kill specific civilizations. The terrestrial and air traffics have multiplied during the last decades. All of these aspects have a profound impact on the spread of infectious diseases, which can be zoonotic or not. Charlatanism, superstitious belief, empiricism may complicate the correct target of contagious diseases. Unfortunately, some journals and newspapers still accept unverified facts and claims, jeopardizing common sense and simple measures to curb epidemics and pandemics.

Ars Medica (τέχνη ιατρική) is crucial because points originate hypotheses, which may be supported by additional facts to consolidate theories. Theories may become common laws or directives, proofing the validity of the scientific process. From Asia Minor and Ionic islands, *Ars Medica* was inspired by pre-Socratic philosophers and Socratic dialectic. Hippocrates of Kos (Ἱπποκράτης ὁ Κῷος, ~460 – ~370 BC) is considered the Father of Medicine and disease. He does not preclude in his oath the pray to Apollo Healer, Asclepius, Hygieia, Panacea, and all the deities, making them his witnesses in practicing medicine. Still, he considered a disease as a natural event instead of a supernatural process. According to the Hippocratic knowledge, our existence is represented by the four essential elements: earth, air, water, and fire, corresponding to four elemental human "*humors*" of blood, phlegm, yellow bile, and black bile. The brain, lung, spleen, and gall bladder were the location of each specific humor, and four "personality" types were identified, including sanguine, phlegmatic, melancholic, and choleric [35]. An imbalance of the four elements may have induced illness. Bloodletting, purging, catharsis, diuresis were used to heal the patient. The blood was considered the most dominant humor by Claudius Galenus of Pergamon (Pergamum, Pergamos) (Κλαύδιος Γαληνό) in the 2nd and 3rd centuries. The practice of venesection has been fulgurated in textbooks and schools [36]. In the 19th century, Louis Pasteur and Heinrich Hermann Robert Koch firmly established the germ theory of disease. The discovery of microscopic pathogens was vital in understanding diseases, and humoral medicine progressively declined. Although Louis Pasteur and Edward Jenner developed the first vaccines to protect against viral infections, the concept of virus was not fully yet there. It seems that the first evidence of the presence of viruses may have originated from experiments with filters that had pores small enough to retain bacteria. In 1892, Dmitri Ivanovsky used one of these filters to show that the juice from a diseased tobacco plant remained infectious to healthy tobacco plants despite being filtered. Martinus Beijerinck called the filtered, infectious substance a "virus," and this discovery is considered the beginning of virology [37]. However, viruses as etiological agents may have already been present in the Chinese wisdom, and the enormous progress in medicine of ancient China is well documented [38-44].

Coronaviruses (CoV) are a broad family of viruses well known to veterinary doctors. CoVs can cause zoonoses, which are infectious diseases caused by a pathogen such as bacteria, viruses, parasites, or prions that suddenly jump from an animal to a human. Zoonosis derives from Greek ζῷον "animal" and νόσος "illness." The transmission of zoonoses entails any context in which there is direct contact with or consumption of animals, animal products, or even animal derivatives. Prominent bacterial examples due to water contamination or food supply include *Escherichia coli*

O157:H7, *Campylobacter*, and *Salmonella* [45-47]. Most influenza virus strains that infect humans are exclusively human diseases, but some swine flu and bird flu strains are zoonoses. These viruses recombine with human strains of the influenza virus, causing pandemics such as the 1918 Spanish flu and the 2009 swine flu [48]. Ebola virus, a microorganism causing a highly lethal hemorrhagic fever, involves chimpanzees, gorillas, orangutans, fruit bats, monkeys, shrews, forest antelope, and porcupines. The transmission mode entails body fluids and organs and emerged in 2013–16, possibly in Africa. Other hemorrhagic fevers (Crimean-Congo hemorrhagic fever, Dengue fever, Lassa fever, Marburg viral hemorrhagic fever, Rift Valley fever) involve camels, rabbits, and hares, hedgehogs, cattle, sheep, goats, horses, and swine. They typically occur through direct contact with infected animals [49]. Two common parasites are associated with the consumption of raw or undercooked meat or seafood. *Echinococcus* commonly affects wild and domesticated animals (wolves, coyotes, foxes, jackals, rodents, and dogs, sheep, as well as pigs) due to the ingestion of eggs from contaminated food water. *Anisakiasis* is due to *Anisakis*, a genus of parasitic nematodes. Larval anisakids are common parasites of marine and anadromous fish (e.g., salmons, sardines). These parasites can also be found in squid and cuttlefish. They are absent from fish in waters of low salinity due to the physiological requirements of krill, a small crustacean, which is involved in the completion of the worm's life cycle. The severe acute respiratory syndrome - coronavirus 1 (SARS-CoV-1) of 2002-2004 started with bats and civets with close contact with humans [50]. The SARS originating in southern China caused 8,098 cases across 37 countries and resulted in 774 deaths. Creutzfeldt-Jacob disease, a prion-based disease (PrPvCJD), is an anti-dogmatic disease associated with cattle eating meat from animals infected with Bovine spongiform encephalopathy (BSE) and occurred worldwide, but mainly in 1996–2001 in the United Kingdom. It is called anti-dogmatic because it entails a transmission from proteins to DNA against the standard way of life reproduction of DNA, RNA, and proteins. Prions are misfolded proteins with this intrinsic ability to spread their misfolded shape onto normal variants of the same protein.

Coronavirus Disease 2019 or COVID-19 is currently a global pandemic that has affected over 200 million people worldwide, resulting in over four million deaths [51-55]. In the last 20 years, several viral epidemics were primarily transmitted by respiratory droplets. The WHO reports that viral diseases continue to emerge and represent a severe threat to public health [56]. Over the last tumultuous 20 years, there have been several viral epidemics, including SARS-CoV-1 from 2002 to 2003, H1N1 influenza in 2009, and MERS-CoV 2012 [56, 57]. Although deadly, they did not reach the extension of damage to human life, economy, and political science as seen in the current pandemic. In December 2019, an unknown disease characterized by pneumonia occurred in Wuhan, the capital of the Hubei Province, China. On January 7, 2020, a novel coronavirus was identified as the agent for the cluster of respiratory illnesses in Wuhan [58-61]. The severe acute respiratory syndrome coronavirus 2 (SARS-CoV-2) causes coronavirus disease 2019 or COVID-19. The SARS-COV-2 shares similarities with SARS-CoV-1 in its genome sequence, biological behavior, and clinical manifestations, although this is not uncommon for coronaviruses. SARS-CoV-2 possesses four major structural proteins: spike surface glycoprotein, small envelope protein, matrix protein, and nucleocapsid protein [62]. It is known that the spike protein binds to host receptors via the receptor-binding domains (RBDs) of angiotensin-converting enzyme 2 (ACE2) [7]. This enzyme is localized in multiple organs other than the respiratory system explaining the variety of symptoms and signs observed during COVID-19. This enzyme may be found in the hemato-lymphoid system, gastrointestinal tract, liver, kidney, and brain. COVID-19 is asymptomatic or entails mild cold symptoms but provokes fever, dry cough, dyspnea, sore throat, rhinorrhea, and dyspnea and is associated with extra-respiratory symptoms, including muscle pain, headache, diarrhea, nausea, and vomiting [5]. A common partial or permanent loss of smell and taste has been associated with COVID-19. In some patients, dyspnea and chest pain can become alarming with severe consequences for respiration and the need for oxygen supply, intubation, or even mechanical ventilation. There is an expected increase in thrombosis. Since the beginning of the pandemic, patients 65 years or older and individuals who suffer from predisposing conditions or disabilities have been considered at high risk. Considering the obesity, overweight, and fatty liver disease identified in Western countries, it is also essential to consider the concomitant factors affecting morbidity and mortality rates. The diffuse use of antibiotics and pesticides in farming and decreased priming of children living in urban centers underexposed to environmental challenges should raise the eyebrows and consider that our immune system is probably weaker than that of our ancestors. Endothelial cells seem not to express ACE2 receptors, but their function is often dysregulated in patients suffering from COVID-19. Typically, this aspect leads to a reduction in lung function. It seems that indirect activation of the endothelium with cell swelling (hypertrophy) results following viral infection, and this change may originate from surrounding tissue damage. This phenomenon seems to be not unusual to viral infections as observed by comparing the lung pathology of deceased individuals affected with other viral infections. The anatomic pathology played a significant role in identifying some histopathology patterns of COVID-19 infection. In patients who suffered from COVID-19, the postmortem investigation of the lung showed extensive lung damage comparable to an acute respiratory distress syndrome or shock lung with significant thrombus formation. The often identified abnormal cells are similar to the cells of other virologic insults to lung tissue. Some of these observations help explain the lingering symptomatology in some patients affected with COVID-19 [62-66]. Although considered a respiratory infection, SARS-CoV-2 can infect various cells, and neurologic symptoms have been described [53]. Also, microscopic investigations of the cardiac cells show structural abnormalities, including severe fragmentation of the sarcomeres and loss of nuclear DNA [67].

The viral spread has been an object of contention among scientists and laypeople. Although stress has been deposited on fomites, a term indicating things or materials likely to carry infection, such as clothes, devices, tools, and furniture, the attention quickly went to respiratory droplets [68-72]. SARS-CoV-2 survives on surfaces, but its longevity and infectivity potential may depend on several factors, including the type of surface, temperature, relative humidity, and specific strains or variants of the virus. There is, however, a large variability, ranging from 2 hours to 9 days [73]. Nevertheless, the virus seems to last on a surface for up to 28 days [74, 75]. Airborne spread is common, which is not unreasonable for respiratory viruses. Initially, it was not acknowledged by most public health organizations, including WHO. In July 2020, after a plea from 239 leading scientists for the airborne spread to be adequately addressed, guidelines were revised to reflect airborne spread as a factor in disease transmission. It seems that ventilation is also crucial to limit the transmissibility of the virus. Some ventilation systems are ancient, not satisfactorily maintained, or ineffective and have been suggested to increase the risk of viral spread, especially in communal spaces. There is a low risk of infection for tears and breast milk and no transmission through mosquitos' bites. Pets are commonly affected with coronaviruses, but these domesticated animals have not been considered a high-risk source of infection. However, some concern is still present that pets may become a "domestic" reservoir spreading the disease to wild mammal populations. Since placental cells minimally express the ACE2 receptor, there are only very few cases and limited evidence of transplacental transmission of SARS-CoV-2 from a mother to her unborn child. Another controversial aspect is the incubation period, which is estimated to be around 5.1 days. Reports suggesting an incubation over this time have not been universally confirmed. Thus, quarantining for 14 days is a helpful recommendation to prevent potential viral spread. Also, testing, which is tackled in the next chapter, remains critical in detecting the live virus in patients who show clinical recovery.

Underlying conditions that may aggravate the course of COVID-19 infection have been delineated. The evidence used to update the list of underlying medical conditions that increase an individual's risk of severe illness from COVID-19 is well reported on the CDC website [76]. Adults of any age suffering from specific primary medical conditions are at increased risk for severe illness from SARS-CoV-2. The CDC specified that severe illness from COVID-19 is defined as hospitalization, admission to the intensive care unit (ICU) with or without intubation or mechanical ventilation, or even death. The use of systematic reviews and meta-analyses support the following primary conditions: cancer, chronic obstructive pulmonary disease (COPD), chronic renal disease, Down (trisomy 21) syndrome, cardiac failure, coronary artery disease, cardiomyopathies, immunocompromised state due to solid organ transplant, obesity (body mass index [BMI] of 30 kg/m^2 or higher but < 40 kg/m^2), severe obesity (BMI ≥ 40 kg/m^2), type 2 diabetes mellitus, sickle cell disease, pregnancy, and smoking. The evidence for the above conditions is decisive. A mixed or moderated proof is provided for some states, including asthma, cerebrovascular disease, cystic fibrosis or mucoviscidosis, hypertension, and prolonged use of corticosteroids and other drugs affecting the immune system. There is limited evidence of a risk for severe illness in the case of a SARS-CoV-2 infection for some conditions. They include immunocompromised state due to blood or bone marrow transplant, immune deficiencies, co- or pre-infection with human immunodeficiency virus (HIV), neurologic disorders, liver diseases, non-COPD lung disease, overweight (BMI > 25 kg/m^2, but < 30 kg/m^2), thalassemic anemia, and type 1 diabetes mellitus. Children are rarely affected. Regarding trisomy 21, researchers found that *TMPRSS2* or Trans-Membrane Protease Serine 2, a gene that cyphers for an enzyme vital for aiding the entry of SARS-CoV-2 in human cells, harbors 60% higher levels of expression in these individuals because the gene is located on chromosome 21. However, the researchers also found signs that people with an extrachromosome 21 have an overactivated interferon response, which is an important innate defensive mechanism that shuts down viral replication within cells. Two more genes – *IFNAR1* (Interferon Alpha And Beta Receptor Subunit 1) and *IFNAR2* (Interferon Alpha And Beta Receptor Subunit 2) – found in the extra chromosome 21, are linked explicitly to the interferon response. These studies strongly advocate for early vaccination protocols for people with the extra-chromosome 21 [77].

CXCL10 or C-X-C motif chemokine ligand 10 is in humans encoded by the *CXCL10* gene, which can trigger the cytokine storm found in COVID-19 patients with severe illness. Several cell types secrete the protein coded by CXCL10 in response to interferon-gamma (IFN-γ) [78]. SARS-CoV-2 induced production in the lung of the pro-inflammatory chemokines and, among them, CXCL10. Also, mRNA for CXCR3, the receptor for CXCL10, was massively expressed in the lungs of SARS-CoV-infected mice [78-80]. *NLRP3* (NOD-, LRR- and pyrin domain-containing protein 3) gene has been critical for maintaining homeostasis against pathogenic infections [55, 81, 82]. The COVID-19 experience in the intensive care unit has been traumatic for both patients and healthcare providers. The burden has been underestimated, raising doubts on the appropriate management of the post-traumatic stress disorders of both patients and healthcare providers. It also indicates how much we deploy to avoid the deterioration of the mental health of healthcare provides. It has been suggested that although COVID-19's effects on the brain have also been examined, most of the psychiatric symptoms seem to be primarily a result of stressful hospital experiences rather than clinical signs unique to COVID-19. On the other side, the role of SAMHD1, a dNTP phosphohydrolase containing the Sterile Alpha-Motif (SAM) and histidine-aspartate (HD) domain, restricts viral replication by limiting the cellular dNTP pool, has been emphasized in COVID-19 infection. SAMHD1 may be the link between SARS-CoV-2 disease, and neurological complications have been the target of intriguing undergoing investigation [53]. The STRING bioinformatic and text mining have associated ACE2 with SAMHD1 and the nuclear factor-kappa B (NF-κB) pathway [53].

Treatment of COVID-19 remains elusive, despite a good understanding that the natural biology of the infection process is critical in determining the most productive and effective treatment. Typically, scientists can focus therapeutics on key targets in preventing virus entry in vulnerable tissues, such as creating a snare version of the ACE2 receptor. In the pathogenesis of COVID-19, there are two main processes in play. An early process is primarily driven by replication of SARS-CoV-2, while a late process is driven by an exaggerated immunologic and inflammatory response to the virus that leads to an irrefragable tissue damage, which can be irreparable. Thus, antivirals are useful early in the course of the disease, while immunosuppressive and anti-inflammatory therapies may play a role in the advanced stages of COVID-19 [83]. Although insufficient data from clinical trials are present, some data suggest that some patients may profit from receiving anti-SARS-CoV-2 monoclonal antibodies early in the course of infection [84]. Currently, *remdesivir*, an antiviral agent, is the only drug that seems to act efficiently and has been approved by the FDA for the treatment of COVID-19 infection. It has been recommended for use in hospitalized patients who require supplemental oxygen [75, 85, 86]. Its use in patients who require mechanical ventilation is not routinely recommended. This decision is due to the lack of satisfactory data showing profiting at this advanced stage of the infectious disease. *Dexamethasone* is a corticosteroid and seems helpful in improving survival in hospitalized patients who necessitate supplemental oxygen. There is direct evidence of benefit for patients who require mechanical ventilation. *Remdesivir* and *dexamethasone* should be given to patients who require increasing amounts of supplemental oxygen. In hospitalized patients requiring oxygen delivery, *dexamethasone* or *dexamethasone* plus *remdesivir* is recommended. If extracorporeal mechanical oxygenation or mechanical ventilation is in place in patients with COVID-19, *dexamethasone* is the only drug recommended by the FDA [83]. Numerous treatments have been proposed in the last 20+ months with positive and negative effects, and some medications have been repurposed [87-90]. Repurposing of drugs is not unusual for anti-cancer or antiviral therapy. However, its politics has been wild and, even excellent medical journals expressed *ad personam* invectives. Following studies on NRLP3 inflammasome [55, 81, 82], probably targeting this inflammasome, i.e., the cytosolic multiprotein oligomers of the innate immune system, which is responsible for the tremendous activation of inflammatory responses, may remain crucial. The cytokine storm can be mitigated following SARS-CoV-2 infection [55]. NLRP3 or NLR Family Pyrin Domain Containing three is a protein. The gene is associated with Muckle-Wells Syndrome and Cinca Syndrome and NLR stands for Nucleotide-binding domain, leucine-rich repeat-containing receptor. This signaling pathway is probably crucial in several inflammatory cascades. In the past, some animal models for inflammatory bowel disease, a chronic inflammatory disease of the gastrointestinal tract affecting both children and adults, and we consider that this target may be crucial to arrest the cytokine storm of patients affected with COVID-19 [82]. The review of the literature seems to indicate that therapy in most of the COVID-19 infections is probably unnecessary because SARS-CoV-2 infection is either asymptomatic or accompanied by mild symptoms. It is important to realize that our aggressive treatment with mechanical ventilation would have been unnecessary. Indeed, only later in the pandemic, it has been demonstrated that early mechanical ventilation may be nocive for numerous individuals, and prone position ventilation has been associated with outstanding results [91]. Lung-protective ventilation, combined with prone position ventilation and adequate sedation and analgesia should remain an essential component of ventilation management in COVID-19 patients [91]. Also, the additional administration of corticosteroids has been associated with better compliance in numerous patients experiencing breathing difficulty.

Animal models are essential in infective diseases. Lucchesi and colleagues contributed to the use of hydroxychloroquine against SARS-CoV-2. They support the role of the NLRP3 inflammasome in the pathogenesis of the respiratory disease [92]. There is enough evidence that the NRLP3 inflammasome is activated in SARS-CoV-2 infection [93]. Acute respiratory distress syndrome (ARDS) with systemic inflammation has a tremendous lung injury associated with the release of inflammatory cytokines IL-6 (interleukin 6) and IL-1β (interleukin 1 beta). A similar cytokine storm is seen in severe SARS-CoV-2 infection [78, 94]. There is a dysregulated pro-inflammatory cytokine cascade. It is triggered by an intense activation of the innate immune response in COVID-19 [95]. Thus, Lucchesi et al. [92] suggested researchers hypothesize that an animal model based on NLRP3 inflammasome may be helpful in COVID-19 [55]. This animal model is used for studying inflammatory bowel disease [81, 82]. *Citrobacter rodentium* is a non-invasive Gram-negative bacterium, which is a natural mouse microorganism. It is often used to study enteric bacteria-induced inflammation [81, 82]. Transmembrane Toll-like receptors-2 (TLR-2) and TLR-4, the signaling adaptor protein myeloid differentiation factor (MyD)-88, and NF-κB mediate the inflammatory response to *C. rodentium* similarly as in the autophagy-inflammasome interplay of heart failure [96]. COVID-19 patients experience gastrointestinal symptoms that may suggest an inflammatory bowel disease, at least in some patients [97, 98]. The intestinal homeostasis and epithelial integrity are intimately regulated [99].

During the activation of the NLRP3 inflammasome, there is procaspase-1 dimerization and self-activation and *C. rodentium* can also induce caspase-1-dependent IL-1b maturation and flow through a synergistic TLR-4 and NLRP3 path *in vivo* [55]. Mice lacking the *Nlrp3* gene are more susceptible to induced experimental inflammatory bowel disease, and Nlrp32/2 macrophages did not respond to pathogen-associated microbial patterns. Alipour et al. previously demonstrated that compensation of IL-1b in mice lacking the NLRP3 inflammasome might promote the clearance of *C. rodentium* by stimulating inflammatory macrophages in the early stages of infection. On the other hand, IL-1b overcompensation may be disadvantageous in wild-type mice [82]. Thus, animal models may be the key to selecting better drugs or drug combinations for COVID-19.

Chapter 2

TESTING AND COVID-19 NATURAL IMMUNITY

ABSTRACT

This chapter presents an appraisal on testing on COVID-19 illustrating antigen- and antibody-based immunoassays and the identification of the viral nucleic acid using polymerase chain reaction. The most modern techniques are briefly commented on. The role of metagenomics in COVID-19 is discussed because of the critical interaction of this infection with co-infections.

Keywords: testing, antigen-based assay, antibody-based assay, polymerase chain reaction, metagenomics, SARS-CoV-2.

Three levels of testing are currently known and practiced for COVID-19. They include antigen-based assays, antibody-based assays, and nucleic acid-based assays. Chinese scientists' rapid sequencing and availability were a pillar for the virus structure to be known worldwide. SARS-CoV-2 was first identified on January 5th, 2020, by a Shanghai Public Health Clinical Center, China. On January 10th, 2020, the novel coronavirus genome was posted publicly for all scientists on virological.org and GenBank to assist investigators worldwide [100]. *Coronaviruses* belong to the *Coronavirinae* subfamily, which is part of the family of *Coronaviridae,* and the subfamily contains four genera, including Alpha, Beta, Gamma, and Deltacoronavirus [101]. The genome of CoVs is a single-stranded positive-sense RNA (+ssRNA) with 27–32 kilobases (kb). The capsid outside the genome is formed by the nucleocapsid protein (N). The viral genome is further packed by an envelope, which is typically associated with three proteins, including the membrane protein (M), spike protein (S), and envelope protein (E). The genome size of SARS-CoV-2 is approximately 29.9 kb [102]. It contains four structural proteins (S, E, M, and N) and sixteen non-structural proteins (nsp 1−16) [101]. There are essential functions associated with some non-structural proteins. Nsp1 facilitates RNA processing and replication, nsp2 alters the survival signaling pathway of the host cell, nsp3 is vital in the separation of the translated protein, and nsp4 contains a transmembrane domain 2 (TM2) and transforms the membranes of the endoplasmic reticulum. Also, nsp5 partakes in the process of polyprotein during replication, while nsp6 contains a transmembrane domain. Nsp7 and nsp8 increase the combination of nsp12 and template-primer RNA. While nsp9 functions as an ssRNA-binding protein, nsp10 is critical for the cap methylation of viral mRNAs. Nsp11 is a 13-amino acid long peptide with apparently unprecise function [103]. Nsp12 contains the RNA-dependent RNA polymerase, which possesses an essential component of coronavirus replication/transcription. At the same time, nsp13 binds with adenosine triphosphate (ATP). Singularly, the zinc-binding domain in nsp13 participates in the process of replication and transcription. Nsp14 is a proofreading exoribonuclease domain, while nsp15 has Mn^{++}-dependent endoribonuclease activity. Finally, nsp16 is a 2'-O-ribose methyltransferase. Following SARS-CoV-2 infection, nsp16 binds mRNA recognition domains of the U1 and U2 snRNAs to suppress mRNA splicing. NSP1 binds to 18S ribosomal RNA in the mRNA entry channel of the ribosome to interfere with mRNA translation. The 7SL RNA attracts both nsp8 and nsp9. The signal recognition particle RNA, also known as 7SL RNA, locates at the signal recognition particle and strikingly acts to disrupt protein trafficking to the cell membrane. Bioinformatic analyses demonstrated that SARS-CoV-2 belongs to the betacoronavirus 2B lineage. It shares about 80% of sequence identity with SARS-CoV-1 [104]. The structure of SARS-CoV-2 was studied with other betacoronaviruses. There is a very close relationship (96% of genomic identity) of SARS-CoV-2 with the bat SARS-like coronavirus strain BatCov RaTG13. This finding seems to support that SARS-CoV-2 has originated from bat coronavirus RaTG13 [105].

Polymerase chain reaction (PCR), a method used to quickly make millions to billions of copies of a specific DNA sample, is at the basis of most tests that are currently offered to diagnose active infection of SARS-CoV-2. This decision relies on the technique's high sensitivity and specificity. In January 2020, the German Center for Infection Research developed the first diagnostic assay as a guideline for diagnosing the virus [60, 106, 107]. Numerous tests have been developed worldwide since then. Several alternative technologies have been developed. They include CRISPR (clustered regularly interspaced short palindromic repeats), loop-mediated isothermal amplification (LAMP), and mass spectrometry, despite their costs was comparable superior to PCR. CRISPR-Cas 9 is both a gene-editing tool and a diagnostic tool [108].

Antibody-based testing is used to detect a previous infection. There is a range of such tests, which have been developed to identify people who have previously been infected. Such tests are helpful because they determine past exposures, detect convalescent plasma donors, and help estimate immunity levels within a population. Such a test can distinguish between early immunoglobulins (IgM) and late immunoglobulins (IgG). It gives crucial information about the phase of infection, indicating how long ago the person was substantially infected with SARS-CoV-2. An antibody-based test can also help to identify the individuals who should be prioritized for vaccinations and, of course, potential donors for convalescent plasma therapy. In July 2020, only around 5% of the Spanish population in Spain, a country heavily hit by SARS-CoV-2, had antibodies against this virus. This percentage is not even close to the levels estimated to be safely required for natural herd immunity. Importantly, this value may not be accurate because some people can ensure a T-cell-mediated immunity to the virus, even they are not detected by antibody tests. It has been indicated that only six out of ten individuals affected with COVID-19 develop protective antibodies towards SARS-CoV-2. Also, the antibody levels towards the virus decline rapidly in the months after the infection, although some memory in the immune system may still be present. Antibody-based testing relies on a laboratory-based assay. Examples are ELISA (enzyme-linked immunosorbent assay), CIA (chemiluminescent immunoassay), or a point-of-care (POC) test. The last test is based on lateral flow technology [109, 110]. Negative results can occur following antibody-based testing if the test is taken too shortly after infection before the body has efficiently produced antibodies. False-positive results may occur due to cross-reactivity of the test with antibodies present due to any previous infection with other coronaviruses. Several antibody tests are commercially available by companies like Roche, Beckman-Coulter, EUROIMMUN, and Abbott. Finally, Verkerke et al. suggested the potential utility of IgA serology in the acute setting. They explored the benefits and limitations of class-specific serology as a complementary diagnostic tool to PCR for COVID-19 in the acute setting. IgM and IgG may disclose a false positivity [111].

Antigen-based testing is a formidable tool to identify if a person is presently infected with SARS-CoV-2, but once the infection has disappeared, the antigen vanishes as well. Contrasting nucleic acid-based tests such as PCR, antigen tests detect proteins or glycans, such as the spike proteins of the virus. The production of such assays can be a complex and time-consuming laboratory process. In addition, accuracy testing is often a problem with such a tool because antigen tests usually have much lower sensitivity than PCR. Advantages are rapid turnaround time, relatively cheap, and more amenable to point-of-care (POC) use. Some of such tests may have been proposed by companies such as Quidel, OraSure, Iceni Diagnostics, and E25Bio [112, 113]. Some pharmaceutical companies have also launched a very rapid antigen diagnostic kit that can quickly detect the presence of SARS-CoV-2 infection within few minutes [110]. Kits have been received emergency use approval from the WHO. They often harbor excellent performance of 90% sensitivity and 96% specificity [112, 113]. However, suppose patient test results positive using such kits. In that case, health authorities will need to proceed with a final determination using a PCR test, which targets the virus's ribonucleic acid. Such rapid antigen diagnostic kits use an antigen-antibody binding reaction by testing a sample collected from the nasal cavity.

Metagenomics and its role in health are being intensely investigated in the last few years. Metagenomics is also known as environmental genomics. Another name is advanced genomics (μετά - is the preposition or prefix derived from the Greek meaning after). Metagenomics collects investigations of genetic material recovered directly from environmental samples. Metagenomics has also been referred to as environmental genomics, eco-genomics or, even community genomics. The potential role of co-infection in aggravating the SARS-CoV-2 infections is heavily debated, but it may help understand the severity of some cases in the young populations. Microbial cell-free DNA sequencing (mcfDNA-Seq) in patients admitted to the ICU with COVID-19 indicates a higher incidence rate of probable secondary diseases than previously recognized. This metagenomic study identified a significant association between mcfDNA and 30-day mortality, suggesting that COVID-19 severity may be influenced by circulating bacterial fragments, either from secondary pneumonia or possible translocation of colonizing microbiota along the disrupted alveolar/epithelial surface of lungs injured by SARS-CoV-2 infection [114, 115]. This data is not trivial and has been confirmed in more recent investigations as well. Vigilance and thorough diagnostic workup in patients with COVID-19 infection of moderate or severe degree and antibiotic use should probably be the main tasks to control the death rate of patients with SARS-CoV-2 disease [114]. Metagenomics can be crucial to trace and manage any outbreak during the COVID-19 pandemic successfully. Virtually all infectious agents contain DNA or RNA genomes, and metagenomic sequencing represents an attractive approach for pathogen detection [116]. The cost of next-generation sequencing (NGS) or high-throughput has been notably reduced since its introduction in 2004. These techniques have emerged as an enabling technological platform for detecting and taxonomic characterizing multiple microorganisms in several clinical samples from different patients. Metagenomics using NGS can detect all organisms in a sample, regardless of whether they are known or novel pathogens and they are single or multiple co-infections. Carbo et al. outlined the validation of a metagenomics protocol for coronavirus identification [117]. The use of centrifuge and genome detective resulted in the assignment of the NGS reads to the closest relatives of the emerging coronaviruses. Capture probes targeting vertebrate viruses, designed in 2015, enhanced both sequencing depth and coverage of the SARS-CoV-2 genome, the latter increasing from 71% to 98%. It provides a potential tool for pandemic preparedness by simulating novel virus discovery [117]. The potential of metagenomics in discovering and tracing novel coronaviruses is enormous.

Pangolins are still sold in wet markets, as pointed out in March 2020 in a Nature paper, and metagenomics may play a crucial role [118, 119]. The metagenome of the host remains a question mark in COVID-19. It may be essential to remember that such a variable may be the underlying condition to understand the variability of the infection of COVID-19. It is also necessary to remember that individuals with fewer sugars in their diet, richer in probiotics, experience fewer symptoms than the typical population [120]. Gut microbiota impacts the spread of pathogens. They control the inflammation response, organ damage, and death of the affected individual. It is well known that commensal microbiota can highly modulate the production of interferon in the lung. This aspect is crucial in the defense not only against SARS-CoV-2 but also against other viral infections, such as the influenza virus [121-123]. It has been demonstrated that about 50% of the general population have a T-cell response to SARS-CoV-2 due to cross-reactivity to common cold viruses [124]. This data can explain the large numbers of asymptomatic carriers of the virus and, potentially, the high degree of variation in the severity of COVID-19.

The innate response is not the unregulated adaptive immune response via T cells that determines morbidity and death in severe COVID-19 [125]. The direct Oxford Nanopore long-read 3rd generation metatranscriptomic sequencing may be critical to evaluate further the response to viruses and vaccines [126]. SARS-CoV-2 surveillance may involve wastewater monitoring, portable and wearable sensors for detecting viruses and bacteria in the surrounding environment. SARS-CoV-2 immunity is crucial to obtain an optimal herd immunity, but we will likely never reach herd immunity against COVID-19. As evinced from the introductory text, the immune system is an essential line of defense in short- and long-term protection from invading pathogens, including SARS-CoV-2. Two components guard the immune system, including innate immunity and adaptive immunity. The body's first line of defense is innate immunity, which provides a rapid but relatively haphazard response against anything that may be considered non-self by the body. On the other hand, the adaptive response of the immune system is a more prolonged but delayed response that reacts specifically to a given threat. It is this response that is substantially responsible for developing long-term immune memory. Specific antibodies and memory B and T cells are included in such a response and protect the organism against future encounters. The organism uses phagocytic neutrophils, macrophages, and dendritic cells to fight against viral infections. However, a potentially lethal overreaction of the immune system response remains critical in understanding the natural history of COVID-19 progression. The "cytokine storm," as often labeled this overreaction, is determined by a buildup of chemokines, proteins used in cellular communication, and immunologic cells. Severe COVID-19 disease has been associated with such an immune system's overactivity. In some patients, underlying disorders and diet influence seem relevant, leading to severe COVID-19 clinical signs. Herd immunity occurs when a satisfactory proportion of the population is alive and has immunity to a given infection. Very variable rates have been presented by eminent immunology experts and politicians, complicating the overall picture for the layperson. We know that herd immunity slows or prevents disease spread, and such action protects "at-risk" individuals. However, even adjuvanted by vaccination, natural infections cannot determine the exact rate of herd immunity that must be reached with safety. Numerous socio-economic, environmental, and genetic variables may play a role. Thus, the wisdom is to avoid spreading panic and rely on facts, and mandatory vaccination may be vital in breaking the pandemic spiral.

Chapter 3

Containment Levels and Preventive Measures

Abstract

Facing a disaster from a human and economic perspective, a pandemic such as the current COVID-19 pandemic raises some obvious discussion points. However,it mainly involves the nature and degree of containment levels. In this chapter, containment levels, lockdown, and facemasks are briefly explained.

Keywords: COVID-19, droplets, facemasks, public health, competency

The whistleblower is an individual (e.g., an employee) who publicizes information or activity within a public, private, or government structure or organization deemed, in good faith, fraudulent, illegal, illicit, unsafe, or abusive. The approach to whistleblowers differs from dictatorial to democratic systems, although exceptions are found in both systems. Typically, despite being considered bad counterintuitively, at least initially, whistleblowers' actions are good for society, mainly if they are structured. Creating a non-toxic environment where employees feel comfortable sharing their concerns and managers evaluating constructive criticisms and responding to them supports a positive culture. Some healthcare whistleblowers in China were flagging on Asian social media, and an unknown infection like a Coronavirus infection seemed to occur only on December 31st, 2019. The first cases of a novel coronavirus were officially identified in Wuhan, the capital of the Hubei Province. After several discussions but without thorough investigation, the initial outbreak of the disease was considered alarming. Still, it was declared a PHEIC (Public Health Emergency of International Concern) by the WHO only on January 30th, 2020. This decision is crucial. Global public health risk of the disease and a coordinated international response were requested. However, some kind of dilettantism was evident since the beginning, considering the WHO approach to policies of facemasks and international travel restrictions. In China, both facemasks and travel restrictions, and strict lockdowns were mostly implemented with spectacular results. Some advocated measures by the director Dr. Ghebreyesus and his team were probably not utterly devoid of ambiguity and inadequate modernization, giving ground to conspiracy theory to proliferate. At the pandemic's beginning, the WHO did not recommend using facemasks and travel bans to control SARS-CoV-2 spread. Substantially, this policy was based on more than a century-old normative practice that recognized such restrictions are precepted leaky to prevent pathogen spread. They may interrupt the flow of essential goods, including medical supplies. Countries such as New Zealand, Australia, and Taiwan have proved the utility of travel restrictions in slowing the spread, giving time for administrations to establish an adequate public health response strategy [127].

Dr. Ghebreyesus, who is an Ethiopian biologist, serves since 2017 as Director-General of the WHO. Despite some criticisms, raised inside the African Union, Dr. Ghebreyesus was successful in obtaining this position. He is the first non-physician in this role to the best of my knowledge. Despite the probably initial inadequate response, preventative measures such as travel restrictions started to be put in place in some countries, such the US. Since then, the disease, currently officially known as COVID-19, has been declared a pandemic, spread to over 200 countries with over 200 million confirmed cases, and claimed the lives of over four million people.

Facemasks were effectively used in Asian countries despite controversial and unsubstantiated WHO statements. The WHO and public health advisers have since advised governments to encourage the use of non-medical face coverings or facemasks amongst the public where physical distancing is not possible. The fear of repercussions against Asian communities brought a heavy politicization of the event. Political correctness was interposed to public health measures. In the early stages of this pandemic, China's response was not marvelous about containing the outbreak. Subsequenty, building efficient containment centers in very few days has been a very good response. The nucleic acid sequence revealed by Chinese investigators allowed other researchers worldwide to set up some testing measures. Inadequate and passive responses of the Chinese governments were demoted, but whistleblowers suffered, and one of them died of COVID-19 [128]. It is important to acknowledge that the rapid presentation and diffusion of data and sequences provided by Chinese agencies and institutions has been vital in accelerating the testing methods. Strict lockdowns and the impressive construction of a COVID-19 hospital in Wuhan have been praised worldwide. Current research indicates that SARS-CoV-2 is re-emerging in many locations following summer 2020 and the relaxation of lockdown restrictions, although several parameters should be taken into account. Diagnostics of COVID-19 is vital and relies on good information about the virus's structure and genetics. The virus was isolated and successfully cultured in virology labs, which scientists in Australia and France achieved in January 2020 outside China [129]. Scientists from The Peter Doherty Institute for Infection and Immunity (Doherty Institute) in Melbourne successfully grown the coronavirus from a patient sample, which provided international expert laboratories with crucial information for testing. At the same time, the virus responsible for the cases of pneumonia that emerged in China was cultured at the Institute Pasteur of France [130]. By February 2020, the complete viral genome had been sequenced. Several SARS-CoV-2 genome sequences were made publicly available for researchers worldwide, and this aspect features the scientific collaboration of the communities independent from the origin. The original consideration of genetic engineering for the source of the virus is currently considered unlikely. Most probably, the virus seems to be a product of natural selection. Lineage genomics support strongly the concept that the virus has been circulating in bats for decades like many other coronaviruses, which can infect humans. Pangolins have been suggested as the potential intermediate host, but more research is still needed. At the time of the pandemic, most of the Chinese wet markets were closed. In the wet market, apart from fresh domestic animals, also wild animals are sold. Since the beginning of the pandemic, numerous variants have been characterized. Still, variants circulating in South Africa, the United Kingdom, Europe, India, and the United States of America considerably increased the virus's capability to infect cells. However, the deadly rate seems to be still controversially discussed.

Safety is a dynamic and learning activity. Once certification is obtained, the process starts to comprehensively evaluate the environment in terms of safety or near-miss incidents. It means that any purpose of safety valid today may not be right tomorrow. The state of being protected (static) and preserved (dynamic) from damage or injuries affects individuals' life, health, and bodily integrity. A series of metrics track the rate of injuries and fatalities and illnesses, and even near misses. A condition to a proper safety level is the thorough investigation of any incident, the correct and periodic performance of drills, and systematic evaluation of metrics involving near misses. While injuries, illnesses, and fatalities are easy to understand, near misses may not be reported, and failing it may trigger a chain reaction and a laxity that may be fatal on a subsequent occasion. Any organization needs to ensure that all safety protocols and measures are constantly being followed, implemented new ones if needed, and performed periodic drills. Although the dread of insane costs for fines is the trigger to follow safety procedures (passive behavior), fulfill and clear explanation of safety measures in periodic training (dynamic behavior) targets the full definition of safety. Regulatory bodies require a variety of actions employers must take. These organizations have the authority to impose fines if their investigations reveal a violation of these standards, which have a stricter application than guidelines. The National Fire Prevention Association (NFPA) advanced a hazard rating system. This standard, NFPA 704, summarizes a hazard rating system ranging from 0 to 4 for emergency personnel. There is a colored section, and a numerical rating is given to the hazard. The system uses a color-coded diamond with four quadrants in which numbers are used in the upper three quadrants. The colors signal the degree of health hazard (blue), flammability hazard (red), and reactivity hazard (yellow). The white bottom quadrant is used to indicate unique risks.

OSHA or Occupational Safety and Health Administration is a significant regulatory agency of the United States Department of Labor. Originally, OSHA had federal visitorial powers to inspect and examine workplaces. Cultivating a safe culture everywhere, both at home and at work takes extensive picture reasoning. Preventing and removing workplace hazards is required for employee safety. Under the Occupational Safety Health Act's General Duty Clause, it is a legal responsibility requiring all employers to provide a free workplace from recognized hazards that may cause severe harm or death to their employees. OSHA's Workplace Hazards are five and include 1) safety, 2) chemical, 3) biological, 4) physical, and 5) ergonomic [131]. OSHA aims always to mitigate employee risk. Safety hazards encompass any substance, condition, or object that can injure workers. Some examples of safety hazards include cords or boxes blocking walkways, spills on floors, falls from heights, machines having moving parts, confined spaces, and electrical hazards such as frayed cords. Chemical hazards may include acids, carbon monoxide, fiberglass fibers, flammable liquids, pesticides, silica dust, and welding fumes. Conversely, biological hazards include some events such as animal droppings, blood, fungi, mold, and viruses. Physical hazards, on the other side,include radiation, heat shock or extreme cold working conditions, constant exposure to loud noise. Ergonomic hazards include working conditions unfavorable for the musculoskeletal system and may consist of repetitive work or work in a particular position straining the body. The Global Harmonized System of Classification and Labeling of Chemicals (GHS) is a method for communicating chemical hazards [132-134]. GHS was developed and propagated by the United Nations (UN) and has been successfully adopted in many countries. Before GHS, countries were each using their labeling system. The lack of international standards and the enactment of international languages, such as English, in standard operating procedures increases remarkably the risk of laboratory accidents. Originally, recipients of chemical shipments could not quickly identify the hazards presented by their packages. The GHS aimed to eliminate this confusion by providing clear guidelines for chemical labeling that can be used across borders. GHS's first edition was issued in 2003. In 2012, OSHA integrated GHS into its Hazard Communication Standard (HazCom). The new regulations are currently being implemented by manufacturers, importers, distributors, and employers mostly worldwide. Although the GHS is not a legal requirement, many countries are adopting these standards because they simplify the transport and storage of chemicals. In conclusion, the elimination of workplace hazards may, at first glance, appear time-consuming or even expensive. Still, in the long term, they help in avoiding lawsuits and permanent illnesses and increase productivity.

Containment levels describe the physical requirements of laboratories [135]. Risk groups refer specifically to the pathogenicity of the organisms. In Biosafety Level 1, the management is set to manage the lowest risk, while Biosafety Level 4 must handle the highest risk to human or animal health. *Biosafety Level 1* involves infectious agents of Risk Group 1 with biological agents that are incongruously to trigger disease in healthy workers or animals, and Containment Level 1 entails no special facilities, equipment, or procedures are required. Basic safe laboratory practices and standard well-designed experimental animal and laboratory facilities are sufficient. Hand-washing facilities and disinfectant solutions have to be provided. In the *Biosafety Level 2*, Risk Group 2, infectious agents can cause human or animal disease. Examples are *Papillomavirus* or *Herpes Simplex Virus* (HSV). Under normal circumstances, it is improbable that they constitute a serious hazard to laboratory workers, the community, livestock, or the environment (moderate individual risk, limited community risk). Laboratory exposures infrequently produce infection leading to serious disease. Effective care and preventive actions are available, and the risk of dissemination is considered limited. Risk Group 2 infectious microorganisms include *E. coli*, *Salmonella*, and several flu viruses. In the setting of biosafety level 2, facilities, equipment, and procedures required to contain risk group 2 organisms at Level 2 entail laboratory separated from other activities, biohazard signs, room surfaces invulnerable and readily manageable (cleaness). Thus, a laboratory with biosafety level 2 should include an autoclave, certified high-efficiency particulate air (HEPA) filtered class I or II biological safety cabinet for organism manipulations. Personal protective equipment (PPE) includes both laboratory coats worn only in the laboratory, and gloves worn when handling potentially infected material and infected animals. Filters meeting the HEPA standards are required to satisfy certain levels of efficiency. Such standards are the necessity to remove—from the air that passes through—at least 99.95% (Europe) or 99.97% (US) of particles whose diameter is equal to 300 nm (0.3 µm) [136]. All contaminated material needs to be properly decontaminated before being transferred. When a laboratory is decommissioned, the safety cabinet may be transferred to another laboratory. *Biosafety level 3* laboratories handle risk group 3 infectious agents, which are pathogens that usually cause serious human or animal disease or result in serious economic consequences but do not usually disseminate by casual contact from one individual to another. Biosafety level 3 handle high individual risk and low community risk agents. Thus, such agents can be treated by adequate antimicrobial or antiparasitic agents. Biosafety level 3 laboratories target risk group 3 pathogens. They include bacteria such as anthrax (*B. anthracis*), Q Fever (*C. burnetii*), tuberculosis (*M. tuberculosis*). They also include hantaviruses, human immunodeficiency viruses, eastern and western equine encephalitis viruses. Biosafety level 3 laboratories include facilities, equipment, and procedures needed to contain risk group 3 organisms. These laboratories must include a specialized design and construction, controlled access with double door entry, proper decontamination body shower, sealed wall penetrations, and ventilation systems harboring negative air pressure. The negative value of air pressure must be maintained in all surrounding areas. Air should not be recirculated, and the air exhausted must harbor a dedicated exhaust or HEPA filtration system. Also, minimum furnishings, all readily cleanable and sterilizable (fumigation) are present. Laboratory windows are sealed and unbreakable. Backup power must be available, and equipment must include an autoclave, certified HEPA filtered class II biological safety cabinet for organism manipulations, and a dedicated hand-washing sink with the foot, knee, or automatic controls near the exit. PPE should include solid front laboratory clothing, which must be worn only in the laboratory, headcovers, special footwear and gloves. Also, appropriate respiratory protection, depending on the infectious agents, needs to be in use. A series of exit procedures should be known to the employees, including showers, depending on infectious agents used and manipulations involved. All animal wastes need to be disposed of as contaminated laboratory materials. Any activity involving infectious materials must be conducted in biological safety cabinets using appropriate PPE and updated physical containment devices. Full training of the laboratory staff in the handling of pathogenic and other hazardous materials is compulsory. Also, laboratory staff must perfectly use safety equipment, disposal techniques, handling of contaminated waste, and appropriate emergency response protocols. Standard Operating Procedures (SOPs) must be provided and posted within the laboratory outlining. SOPs must contemplate operational protocols for waste disposal, disinfection procedures, and appropriate emergency response protocols. In the facility, it should be a medical surveillance program appropriate to the agents utilized. Finally, a laboratory of *Biosafety Level 4* addresses risk group 4 infectious agents are pathogens that usually produce profoundly serious human or animal diseases, which are often without current treatment. The microbiological agent may be readily transmitted from one individual to another, animal to human or vice-versa directly or indirectly, alternatively, by casual contact, i.e., we are in the presence of high individual risk and high community risk. Microorganisms that belong to the risk group 4 are all viruses, such as Ebola viruses, Foot and Mouth Disease, and Herpes B virus (Monkey virus). In this setting, containment level 4 is the highest level of containment. It is characterized by a remote unit that is completely self-contained to function independently. There is a high level of specialization. There is an airlock for entry and exit. Class III biological safety cabinets or positive pressure ventilated suits are present. Also, a separate ventilation system with full controls to contain contamination needs to be provided. It is paramount to stress that only fully trained and authorized personnel may enter any level 4 containment laboratory. Importantly, on exit from the area, laboratory personnel must shower and re-dress in street clothing. Any microorganisms manipulations have to be performed in class III biological safety cabinets or in conjunction with a one-piece, positive-pressure-ventilated suit [136].

Lockdown or quarantine are two often words we have constantly heard since March 11, 2020, when the WHO formally recognized the global spread of SARS-CoV-2 infection as a pandemic [104, 137]. Quarantine refers to the separation of sick people with a contagious disease from healthy individuals in various ways. This separation is considered as forced segregation in a specific environment or country to prevent the infectious disease from spreading [138]. The Italian word '*Quarantena*,' which means 40 days, and the corresponding Latin word '*Quadrāgintā*' is at the origins of the English word [18, 139]. As tragically depicted by Boccaccio in quarantined people, during the 14th century, 40 days was the length of strict isolation required for ships suspected of carrying an infectious or contagious illness before crew and passengers could land. The Venice Republic suffered from the Black Death enormously. Venice mandated the '*Quarantena*' to any travelers. Quarantine entered the English language in the early 1600s [19, 140]. According to the current knowledge, the bubonic plague has an average 37-day period from infection to death [18]. Thus, the European quarantines would be highly successful in determining crews' health from potential trading and supply ships, but quarantine acquired a religious connotation soon [21]. Despite Hippocratic and Galen reasonings, the disease was often associated with sins. In the Bible, 40 days is found as a period of purification for illness and puerperal rest, but also the Universal Flood was for 40 days and 40 nights. Moses stayed on Mt. Sinai for 40 days. Jesus fasted. In this time, Jesus was tempted by the devil in the desert for 40 days. In human history, quarantine was declared many times following the Black Death, and particularly when infectious disease threatens the population of a town, region, or country. Unlike the early use of lockdown in Europe, the development of a national quarantine policy entered society in America or Canada later. On the origin, the single federal states were responsible for handling the entry of infectious illnesses. The first quarantine station and hospitals in the United States were built in 1799. It was located at the port of Philadelphia, Pennsylvania. It occurred after a yellow fever outbreak in 1793. However, repeated epidemics of yellow fever revealed some failure to contain the spread of infectious diseases. In 1878, Congress released the National Quarantine Act creating the premises for a federal engagement [141]. In 1892, a cholera outbreak led public officials to issue more authority imposing strict requirements, and, eventually, in 1921, the 'quarantine system' was nationalized. The Public Health Service Act established the federal government's Quarantine Authority in 1944. The Centers for Disease Control and Prevention (CDC) instituted the National Communicable Disease Center, which took over federal quarantine functions, in 1967. In the '70s, CDC reduced the number of quarantine stations from 55 to 8 because infectious diseases were thought a relic of ancient history. Still, the number of quarantine stations increased to 20 between 2004 and 2007 because of fears and concerns about bioterrorism after the World Trade Center attack in 2001, and the worldwide spread of disease after the SARS-CoV-1 outbreak in 2003 [142]. Quarantine refers to people who have neither signs nor symptoms but are potentially exposed to a communicable disease. Quarantine needs to be kept separated from isolation. The latter term indicates a separation of symptomatic people or individuals who are reasonably believed to be infected with a contagious disease, separating them from those who are not infected [18, 142]. Recently, our group has developed a computational model rooted in the physics of fluids, aiming to predict the fitness landscape of the COVID-19 virus diffusion using a variant of the bidimensional Ising model connected seasonally. Markov chain Monte Carlo method identifies that an increase in temperature proves a reduced virus diffusion, while increased mobility leads to increased virus diffusion [31].

Facemasks are a method to limit the spread of infectious disease and, despite there may be a straightforward understanding about the usefulness of such simple measure, has been a contentious argument for most of the time of this pandemic polarizing families, races, political parties, and the whole society [51, 69]. The primary source of infection in COVID-19 remains unknown, but the human-to-human transmission was noticed early after the rise of the pandemic. Genomic analysis of SARS-CoV-2 was rapidly shared with the extensive scientific community by Chinese scientists. It shows a phylogenetical relationship of SARS-CoV-2 to SARS-like viruses. At the onset of COVID-19, the most common symptoms are fever, cough, and fatigue [57, 58], while other symptoms may include hemoptysis, dyspnoea, headache, and lymphedema [57, 58]. As identified in several clinical reports, severe COVID-19 cases can progress to pneumonia, which is more or less rapidly accompanied by multi-organ failure and subsequent death. Typically, 97.5% of people will probably develop clear symptoms within 12.5 days of infection, but the asymptomatic period could last up to 14 days, or even 28 days [56, 61, 143]. Epidemiological data indicate that pre- and asymptomatic individuals can also propagate the coronavirus. Asymptomatic individuals may play a significant role in the pandemic. Considering this aspect, a portable device able to detect the virus instantly may be crucial in the future to inexorably stop any epidemics or pandemic. Like other respiratory microorganisms, the transmission of SARS-CoV-2 occurs through aerosol droplets from sneezing and coughing [56, 57]. The primary reproductive number, R_0, relies on epidemiological data. It identifies the exponential growth rate of a specific outbreak. Additional factors may influence this number. The latent period and the infectious period are probably two important key factors. The R_0 seems to have been fluctuating and quite different from what has been calculated originally (2.2-2.7). Some authors found a frightening R_0 of 5.7 with a relatively broad 95% CI (3.8–8.9) (CI, confidence intervals) [144]. This value may better enlighten the pandemic dissemination intially than an R_0 of about 2.5. However, some more recent calculations suggest around 2 or even lower now (about 1.2) that the number of vaccinated people has increased. It has been associated with the hiccups of lockdowns and the occurrence of variants of concern. The use of face masks has been demonstrated to protect healthcare workers as they perform their duties effectively. Still, original data gave limited evidence about whether the everyday use of facemasks was believed to help shield the general population. Although it would be reasonable and cautionary to use facemasks or cloth masks, most public officials opted to be adverse toward their use, primarily due to the hesitancy or ambiguity of the WHO. However, the general population's widespread implementation of wearing facemasks is challenging due to various factors that will be examined later. The extensive use of cloth masks combined with other measures such as social distancing and hand-washing would have potentially reduced the risk of transmission of any virus, including SARS-CoV-2, in January or February 2020 [51, 69].

Infodemic is the side effect we inevitably experienced during this pandemic. Since the declaration of the COVID-19 pandemic, a lot of data has invaded our lives. The inflation of such data and their conflicting findings at the beginning of the pandemic, caused us to be frantic about the correct course of action [145]. Although the application of physical distancing has been primarily accepted worldwide, the level of enforcement was variable and still varies in each country ranging from voluntary to strict legal measures [146]. The overwhelming stress and level of danger that frontline healthcare workers are subject to in this pandemic as they perform their duty to serve the public has triggered great questions. It is a excruciating query of whether they are just a resource that can be exploited, exhausted, and used up [147]. During this pandemic, numerous healthcare workers in the world have died. Many have committed suicide in a tragedy that has touched all continents [148, 149]. The need to increase the efforts in protecting healthcare workers was constant, but the infrastructure and the response have been quite variable during the current pandemic [22, 150-152]. A common view is icons of people wearing masks in public diligently. Face masks have been prevalent in Asian countries since the outbreak of COVID-19, but also before with other outbreaks [69, 153]. In China, some provinces and even municipalities have enforced obligatory mask-wearing in public. However, with spectacular results, China's national guidelines have recommended a risk-based approach for mask-wearing among healthcare workers and the general public [153]. The current dynamics of the COVID-19 pandemic strongly imply human-to-human transmission, which has elicited a humanitarian and economic disaster worldwide [56]. The WHO, which has been a fantastic and prestigious leader in blocking several epidemics effectively in the past, recommends social (physical) distancing, social isolation, and regular hand washing or hand sanitization using an alcohol-based rub in addition to facemasks [154]. However, the WHO has not recommended wearing face masks by the general population until June 5th, 2020 [155]. The CDC advised that persons wear cloth masks in situations where physical distancing would be challenging to maintain. Still, it would have been different if the facemasks or simply face cloths were embraced worldwide early in the pandemic [156]. We had to support cautious advice as the spread of COVID-19 was rapidly increasing. We failed to understand that the death toll was rising, particularly in vulnerable layers of our societies.

Preventive measures in the community are essential to stopping the spread of COVID-19. The most effective preventive measures are still washing hands with soap and water. However, the WHO has no excuse for the missed competency and delayed response in public health, despite some historical considerations [154]. The national recommendations about the use of a face mask for the public vary among countries. Interstingly, the general public uses a range of masks, including cloth masks, dust masks, surgical masks, and N95 masks. In reviewing the chronology of the deployment of the preventive measures despite the COVID-19 pandemic, it seems to be obvious that a certain degree of ambiguities in statements generated a loss of confidence in the public. This ambiguity is probably at the root of some vaccine hesitancy. Uncertainty, and a decision maker's response to it, can be patterned formally in the framework of a general decision model [157]. Both ambiguity and ambiguous attitudes may have a very detrimental effect on some individuals and entire countries have shown a delay in starting a prompt action with deleterious consequences. Surgical masks and N95 masks are considered critical supplies and the CDC advises that they should be reserved for use by healthcare workers who are at a higher risk, but cloth masks or even dust masks or, even increasing the ventilation of rooms, decrease the virus transmission. Face masks combined with other preventative measures such as social distancing and regular hand washing can still play a crucial role in reducing the spread of any virus, including SARS-CoV-2 and its variants [153, 158]. Wearing a face mask in public may have avoided the spread of infectious diseases, including COVID-19, by preventing inhalation and exhalation and, most importantly, the dissemination of contagious droplets [153]. While it is established that airborne droplets carry COVID-19, there is some dispute about the distance that these airborne droplets can travel. Researchers at the Massachusetts Institute of Technology (MIT) in Cambridge, Massachusetts, USA, showed that coughs could project liquid up to 6 meters away under laboratory conditions. Concurrently, sneezes can even allow fluids to travel up to 8 meters [159, 160]. Some experts indicate that the virus can be disseminated by either talking or breathing. It can linger in the air and on surfaces hours after being expelled [159]. Face masks wearing in public can prevent pre-symptomatic persons from transmitting the virus [158]. Even though there are advantages to the general population wearing face masks, there are also disadvantages. In fact, persons wearing masks may become complacent and not adhere to the other recommendations, such as hand washing and physical distancing. Facecloths may be an alternative to facemasks, particularly in time of high demand. In this pandemic, some individuals or countries have stockpiled N95 respirators or facemasks. These unscrupulous people have increased the prices by decreasing the number of products available in the market. Bin-Reza et al. conducted a study that was conducted between November 2009 and January 2011 [161]. This meta-analysis included 17 published randomized control trials and quasi-experimental and observational studies [161]. This meta-analysis was unable to determine a convincing relationship between the use of face masks and protection against influenza or other respiratory infections. It may have jeopardized wise decisions on the beginning [161]. However, Jefferson et al. conducted a review investigating how physical barriers would interrupt or reduce the dissemination of respiratory viruses [162]. The meta-analysis of six case-control studies demonstrated that surgical masks and N95 masks were highly effective in preventing the spread of SARS-CoV-1. The intervention efficacy for frequent hand-washing, wearing a mask, wearing an N95 mask, carrying gloves, dressing in a gown, and hand-washing, mask, gloves, and gown combined was 55, 68, 91, 57, 77, and 91%, respectively [162]. The study concluded that while the enactment of physical barriers could be difficult, these barriers can reduce respiratory infections in the population [163]. Davies et al. directed a study that examined homemade masks as an alternative to commercial face masks. These scientists used healthy volunteers. They compared the efficacy of homemade masks made from cotton, surgical masks, and no masks on their capacity to stop bacterial and viral aerosols [164]. Surgical masks were three times more effective in avoiding microorganisms than homemade masks. Further, 100% of the cotton was the best material to use for homemade masks. Theoretically, breathing constantly synthetic material may be detrimental to our lungs. However, homemade cloth masks have been suggested to be considered a last resort to prevent droplet spread from infected individuals ultimately. Still, homemade cloth masks were considered better than no protection [164]. There are potential challenges to the enactment of widespread face masks in the general population. Unless this order is mandatory, persons would have a choice whether to adhere to this recommendation. Sim et al. stated that individuals are more likely to wear facemasks due to the disease's perceived vulnerability and severity [165]. Taylor et al. determined that youth are less inclined to comply with wearing face masks than older persons. It seems that married individuals are more keen to wear face masks than singles or separated [166]. Also, women are more likely to wear face masks than men. Simultaneously, some cultures and ethnic groups are more prone to wear facemasks than others [166]. While face masks would play an essential role in decreasing the dissemination of any virus, conformity would be tough on the overall outcome unless a mandatory order is in place. Discordant, inaccurate, and ineffective findings lead to confusion among healthcare administrators inciting fake news. Bae et al. studied the effectiveness of surgical and cotton masks in four patients [167]. This article is flawed and has been retracted but has generated false reports [168]. The authors did not fully recognize an important concept, i.e., that of limit of detection (LOD) of the in-house carried out reverse transcriptase-polymerase chain reaction (RT-PCR). They indicated 2.63 log copies per mL, failing to express the values below LOD. Later, comments from readers and scientists worldwide were added to the original publication of the prestigious journal of Annals of Internal Medicine. Bizarrely, the researchers who published in this journal revealed a 36-fold reduction to be "ineffective." We and others disagree. Remarkably, the editors decided to retract the article [168]. Obviously, there is and there will be a debate about solid evidence that face masks can provide adequate protection in the broad community. On the other side, face masks are an important PPE item. They are widely used in medical settings by healthcare professionals during a wide range of medical procedures and practices. As healthcare staff uses both N95 and surgical masks as shields against airborne diseases, it is realistic to think these masks would protect the public worldwide. The public would also require to be constantly educated about the correct way of putting on, wearing, taking off, and disposing of face masks for this to be effective (donning and doffing procedures). At several points of this pandemic adequate instructions were missing. Social media may help achieve the level of understanding for the general population. Finally, the use of cloth masks would deliver an extra layer of protection while preserving the stocks of N95 and surgical masks for healthcare employees and people diagnosed with COVID-19.

R_0 is a parameter that indicates how contagious an infectious disease is. Historiography should consider investigating the late decision to ban non-essential air/land/sea travel in many countries. Also, COVID-19 patients are most infectious in the early days of the disease [144]. It has been calculated that wearing a simple cotton mask will reduce the number of viruses transmitted to a neighbor 36 times [167]. In mathematical terms, if most people wear a mask in public at any time, the transmission rate can quickly decrease beneath 1.0, thus stopping the spread of the disease. The number of COVID-19 cases in South Korea started dropping in February 2020, when the government supplied facemasks to every citizen. In contrast, the number of cases in Italy continued to climb in the same period where facemasks were not provided freely [169]. It is important to emphasize that while a protective mask may reduce the likelihood of infection, it will not eradicate the risk, particularly when a disease has more than one transmission route as identified in SARS-Cov-2. In a situation where there is a short supply of PPE, an improvised facemask should be viewed as the last possible alternative if a commercial product is not available. In China, Hong Kong, Taiwan, Japan, South Korea, and Thailand, the broad assumption is that anyone could be a carrier of the virus. Even seemingly healthy people lead to terrific results in these countries with the widespread wearing of facemasks. Public acceptance of using facemasks in these countries may be attributed to their experience of facing several epidemics. To a certain extent, pollution has triggered facemasks for protection in these countries [170]. Although the pandemic seemed slightly contained, the emergence of fatigue and new variants of SARS-CoV-2 may jeopardize the initial success in numerous countries [171]. The filtration against particles of a size of 3 micrometers performs at 70%. With the spread of the new variants, this efficiency may drop. However, the greater the filtration, the less comfortable the mask is to wear. It may determine an increase in reluctance to wear masks, which is quite understandable.

China's measures for prevention have been mostly fabulous despite initial failure in suppressing whistleblowers in an event that let people remind of the 1986 nuclear accident in Chernobyl and the botched response of the Soviet Union. Apart from these criticisms, the response to the pandemic was good, but this has been a matter of political content without proper historical knowledge. Giving attempts to ridicule the efforts of the Chinese government is not fair, but identifying areas of improvement may be necessary for the whole world. Since ancient times, China has reached a powerful experience in preventing and curing infectious diseases [172]. The Warring States period (475-221 BC) was a period of consolidation of the Chinese empire characterized by military, bureaucratic, and warfare reforms. The Warring States period followed the Spring and Autumn period and concluded with the Qin wars of conquest. The Qin Dynasty annexed all other contender states, which led to the first unified Chinese empire in 221 BC, known as the Qin Dynasty. During the Warring States period, some theories on infectious and epidemic diseases took place in academic circles. In the Qin Dynasty, an integrated response system, including prevention, diagnosis, and isolation, was implemented. Although key concepts were grasped in the Song Dynasty, they gain popularity during the Ming and Qing Dynasties. China was far from understanding biosafety or prevention systems concepts, but in the middle and late Qing Dynasty, remarkable advances in science took place. This period is characterized by a florid exchange of information with missionaries and overseas fellows. During the

Republican period, China developed a modern public health and epidemic prevention system. After founding the People's Republic of China, this country strengthened the biosafety prevention and control system concepts and finally implemented the "prevention first" policy. Of course, there have been weaknesses, and one of the major problems was miscommunication between WHO officials and the Chinese government. It is difficult to identify how it happened, but communication failures are often behind human-made catastrophes and being proficient in English may be a challenge. Tigray's People Liberation Front is the party of Dr. Ghebreyesus, and his political affiliation has been of concern worldwide. It has raised several conspiracy theories during the current pandemic and how WHO handled the initial reaction to the Chinese outbreak by not only praising it, but also profusing reverence at official meetings. The value of disclosing conflicts of interest is still a problem for some public agencies, although private institutions do not usually pledge the disclosure of conflicts. Apart from raising conspiracy theories, the lack of disclosure of conflicts of interest increases public trust's erosion. More than one million signatures were collected to remove Dr. Ghebreyesus from office worldwide. However, Time magazine included him as the 100 Most Influential People of 2020. Still, questions about his candidacy surfaced online, with more than one million people signed in a short time asking for his resignation [173-176]. Although the WHO declared the COVID-19 outbreak a Public Health Emergency of International Concern (PHEIC) on January 31^{st,} 2020 [90], Dr. Ghebreyesus stated there was no reason to limit trade or travel with China. Also, Dr. Ghebreyesus reiterated per WHO and international guidelines that governments adopt policies to stop the spread of the disease that was "evidence-based and consistent" and not to "unnecessarily interfere with international travel and trade." It is critical that future generations re-examine COVID-19 pandemic data and peruse with transparency and honesty the potential misconduct and conflicts of interest of official organizations.

Chapter 4

FACE-/HEAD COVERING AND FAITH

ABSTRACT

In this chapter, we present the importance of face-covering in some faiths. Face-covering is an aspect seen exclusively in several religions and beliefs. It is often seen as an act of reverence and modesty toward the Divinity.

Keywords: belief, face covering, faith, religion

Genesis is the first book of the Torah and the Christian Old Testament. In Genesis 24:63-65, a significant sentence indicates how vital the covering is. We read "*…and Isaac went out to meditate in the field in the evening, and he lifted his eyes and looked, and there, the camels were coming. Then Rebekah lifted her eyes, and when she saw Isaac, she dismounted from her camel, for she had said to the servant, "Who is this man walking in the field to meet us?" The servant said, "It is my master." So, she took the veil and covered herself.*"

63 καὶ ἐξῆλθεν Ισαακ ἀδολεσχῆσαι εἰς τὸ πεδίον τὸ πρὸς δείλης καὶ ἀναβλέψας τοῖς ὀφθαλμοῖς εἶδεν καμήλους ἐρχομένας

64 καὶ ἀναβλέψασα Ρεβεκκα τοῖς ὀφθαλμοῖς εἶδεν τὸν Ισαακ καὶ κατεπήδησεν ἀπὸ τῆς καμήλου

65 καὶ εἶπεν τῷ παιδί τίς ἐστιν ὁ ἄνθρωπος ἐκεῖνος ὁ πορευόμενος ἐν τῷ πεδίῳ εἰς συνάντησιν ἡμῖν εἶπεν δὲ ὁ παῖς οὗτός ἐστιν ὁ κύριός μου ἡ δὲ λαβοῦσα τὸ θέριστρον περιεβάλετο)

Objections to face-covering have been mounting since the start of this pandemic, it is believed. Face mask opponents have been denouncing this public health rule in other pandemics or epidemics as well. It has roots in the face's misidentification that jeopardizes a safe environment for our natural brain processes. A Swiss referendum voted against the face or head covering because it has been associated with Muslim extremists. However, protecting the head or the face has been practiced in other religions as well. As an act of modesty, Rebekah, approaching Isaac, descended from her camel, took the veil, and covered herself. The example of Rebekah in Genesis is emblematic of using a veil as a sign of modesty in approaching people. The marriage of Rebekah to Isaac has brought forward some standard practices. It has been institutionalized in the traditional ceremony of a Jewish wedding. Both bride and bridegroom take part in the "*Badeken*" or "*Bedekung*" (Hebrew/Yiddish: באַדעקן, "covering") ceremony or veiling. Two escorts lead the bridegroom to the bride, and seeing her, the bridegroom covers her face with a veil, like how Rebekah covered her face in approaching Isaac. At this time, the Rabbi pronounces a blessing upon the couple. The bride wears this veil until the conclusion of the chuppah ceremony, which is the time a Jewish couple stand up during their wedding ceremony with a canopy on the top of their heads and extended over four poles by four attendants to the ceremony (Hebrew: חוּפָּה, "canopy"). This tradition with the custom of a virgin bride wearing a veil is mentioned in the Talmud (Ketubot 17b, Rashi ad loc).

Headcovering is also seen in Christian wedding ceremonies, and female attendants in the Moravian Church serving bread to fellow members during the celebration of a love-feast wear head-coverings. In the Hutterite Church (*Hutterische Brüder*), a communal ethnoreligious branch of Anabaptists, wear their head-covering daily. Its remotion takes place only before sleeping. Amish, Hutterites, and Mennonites track their roots to the Radical Reformation of the early 16th century. Jacob Hutter, the founder of the Hutterites, established these communities in 1528 with principles of nonresistance. Although considered inevitably destined to disappear, communities received several tribulations and came from a few hundred to about 50,000 currently. Their practice has been immortalized in several movies, of which the 1985 American movie entitled "Witness" with Harrison Ford is probably harboring one of the most famous screenplays. Currently, almost all Hutterites live in Western Canada and the upper Great Plains of the United States. Head covering was once very common in Orthodox and Roman Catholic churches. Women of Anglican, Lutheran, Calvinist, and Methodist churches were also wearing it. Martin Luther, the Protestant Reformer, urged wives to wear a veil in public worship similar to the veil used by Catolic women. Modesty was a paramount virtue. Christians seem to associate head covering with the tradition found in interpreting the apostle Paul's epistle to Corinthians (1 Corinthians 11:2-6) [177]. In this letter, the Apostle exhorts Corinthians to follow origination and subordination. These two qualities are associated with the headship. The Apostle enlightens that the use of head-coverings is related to God's glory during times of prayer and prophesy. Conscientiously, the author reflects on the Torah usage, and, at the same time, he reconnects Corinthians to Herodotus, an ancient Greek geographer and historian [177, 178]. There is the subordination of Christ to God as the "agent" of Creation. Head covering was universally accepted in Early Christianity. In his texts, Clement of Alexandria, an early theologian of the 1st and 2nd centuries, indicates that the head should be veiled. The face should be covered to avoid the beauty of a woman may become a snare to men [177]. Another Christian Father of the Proto-Christianity of the 1st and 2nd centuries, Tertullian, confirms that Corinthians still wore their veils about one and half centuries after the Apostle addressed them in his epistle. Both Hippolytus of Rome and Origen of Alexandria between the 2nd and the 3rd century confirm this tradition of Proto-Christianity. Subsequently, head covering is still emphasized in the 2nd half of the 3rd century by Victorinus, another Church Father, in his commentary of the Apocalypse of John and, in the 4th century, by John Chrysostom. He stressed that God dictated head-covering [179]. Later, Jerome (347–420) and Augustine of Hippo (354–430) underlined the importance of this tradition. Also, historiography is supported by Early

Christian art. Head covering, both in public and during religious functions, remained common until at least the 18th century for Christian women in European, Mediterranean, Middle Eastern, and African societies. The head covering continues to be practiced in Asia and Africa but is mostly abandoned among contemporary Christians in Europe and North America. Close to the Dalmatian coast, Albanian Christian women often wear white veils, but their eyes are still visible. Indian and South Korean Catholic women still wear the head covering. On the other side, Eastern Orthodox women in Greece show a gradual decline of head covering over the 20th century. In the Catholic Code of Canon Law of 1917, it is indicated that head-covering is mandatory and clothing, which entails prescriptions for both men and women, should be modestly dressed [180]. Veiling was not explicitly referred in the 1983 revision of the Code of the Catholic Church. In the United States, head-covering can vary depending on the congregation's origin, community's denomination, and spread of modernistic or liberal views. Also, the three "John" of the Protestant Church were pro-veil. John Calvin, the founder of the Reformed Churches, John Knox, the founder of the Presbyterian Church, and John Wesley, the founder of Methodism, all reinforced head-covering in public worship [181]. In the United Kingdom, it is still common for women to wear a Christian head-covering (later a bonnet or a hat) while attending formal religious services [182]. Women of Moravian churches, Churches of Christ, Pentecostal Churches, traditional Catholics, Holiness Christians, Laestadian Lutheran Church, Plymouth Brethren, Scottish and Irish Presbyterian, and Dutch Reformed churches have still head-covering. Although not exhaustive, this practice is also observed in women of the Church of Our Lord Jesus Christ of the Apostolic Faith and Jehovah's Witnesses [183]. Also, nuns of the Roman Catholic and other Christian faiths often wear a veil as a part of their religious routine. In the Christian Coptic, head- and face-covering goes over the religious services by stressing this habit in public and the presence of men. During the 19th century, upper-class urban women of Christian and Muslim faiths in Egypt wore *harabah* and *burqa* [62]. As indicated above, head-covering it was and probably should be interpreted in conjunction with modesty in clothing. Decency and propriety belong to modest clothing, which has been stressed over centuries for both men and women. An adequate attire is crucial in any situation in our society, from office to physical activity. Interestingly, head-covering was considered a standard, universal Christian symbolic practice over centuries, despite Christian churches being scattered geographically and containing various cultures. Despite the heavy debate, face or head covering remains a crucial point of reverence in places of worship. It may also be classified as a sign of modesty independently from the religion or belief is practiced. On the other hand, it must be stressed that the face or head covering does not represent a sign of modesty if the practice of either religion or belief is not carried out with sincerity and honesty. Bigotry is never close to God no matter which religion or belief is practiced.

Face masks can be challenging in the long term. The current Face masks have been a challenge for many Christians and many religious people of other believes and confessions. Functions have been terminated, and churches, as well as synagogues and mosques, closed down. We have seen an increased number of spiritual people having difficulty accepting face masks and several religious people supporting anti-mask protests and anti-lockdown or anti-gatherings. In Genesis 1:26-27, the Lord said, "*Let Us make man in Our image, according to Our likeness . . . So God created man in His image; in the image of God He created him; male and female He created them.*" Both males and females of humankind have been created as God's "image" and "likeness". Thus, Lord's image may be "quite" similar to humankind's image. In Christian theology, God is one. Still, three and all (*Deus est trinus et unus et omnia in omnibus*) and God's personification is a human person, i.e., Jesus Christ. There is much emphasis on the face as the epicenter in Genesis, but not the hypocenter of God's glory. In Matthew's description of Christ's transfiguration (Matthew 17:2) [184], Jesus is transfigured before them, and His face shone like the sun with His clothes became as white as the light. Also, in the Song of Solomon 2:14, the sentence is repeated: "Let me see your face, Let me hear your voice; For your voice is sweet, And your face is lovely." Moreover, promiscuity has been associated with face-covering. At the same time, romantic love requires a face visual approach, as expressed in the words, "*When Judah saw her, he thought she was a harlot, because she had covered her face.*" [185]. In the New Testament, the Apostle reports on his epistle to Corinthians (3:17-18): "*Now the Lord is the Spirit; and where the Spirit of the Lord is, there is liberty. But we all, with unveiled face, beholding as in a mirror the glory of the Lord, are being transformed into the same image from glory to glory, just as by the Spirit of the Lord*" [185]. The reaction of many Christians to face masks is the dehumanization associated with it. According to Arnold, authorities with face masks mandates perduring for months are depriving us of Lord's glory. It may be crucial to think that if the world had reacted on time and deceptively, the spreading of this virus would have been limited, and the time of face masks use would have been limited in time. As will be explained in the next chapter, face masks are troubling many people because they fail our capacity to organize our neighbor's image. However, masks are also used by criminals and terrorists concealing themselves during crimes [185]. A plastic shield may be offered instead of face masks, and psychologically and theologically could be compatible, but it probably does not stop the spread of the virus. However, there is another argument that we may consider from a biblical point of view [186]. In chapter 8, the Apostle tells the believers there is no problem eating meat sacrificed to idols because the meat is meat, but not everyone has this knowledge, and we should not create scandal in the eyes of our neighbors. Some of them have been so used to idolatry that when they eat food sacrificed to an idol, their weak conscience is tainted. When we sin like this against brothers and sisters who do not have the full knowledge, we will wound their weak conscience, and we are sinning against the Lord. Therefore, if food triggers my brother or sister to fall, I will never again consume meat so that I will not cause my brother or sister to fall. The same situation is eating pork meat in front of Jewish or Muslims. It is not a sin, but doing it in front of them will necessarily be seen as disrespectful and let their sin because they will hate us. Substantially, the Apostle is telling the church at Corinth to give up their freedoms if they hinder people from coming to Jesus. In practice, wearing the face masks and not eating pork meat is charitable in connection with our neighbors. We live in a community, and our community is not only our church but the humankind.

Chapter 5

VILLAINY AND ANTI-MASK PSYCHOLOGY

ABSTRACT

This chapter presents the history of prejudices and the rise of face coverings in western-styled Hollywood movies and bandits. We highlight the feeling of villainy suscitated by face covering and the misunderstanding of law-abiding people in using facemasks regularly and adequately. The anti-mask psychology has roots that go well further our human understanding. The strong beliefs of anti-mask movements are often misunderstood and dismissed as far-right, but there is anti-mask psychology that needs to be investigated appropriately.

Keywords: Prejudice, face masking, psychology

Wearing a mask is tricky. It may result in a contest when we celebrate Mardi Gras, Halloween, or Birthday parties. Wearing a mask brings a kind of anonymity and, at the same time, get a license to be different or libelous. A cover has been an integral part of some celebration days or "*fasti*" in Ancient Rome, but it is also part of other cultures, such as Asian cultures. However, having a mask continuously de-identify the individuum. It neutralizes our sense of community and sociality. Thus, this chapter starts from a different perspective, showing why people may always feel threatened in masks. It has been suggested that demographic factors such as sex/gender, income level, and political affiliation have been associated with wearing a mask and practicing social or physical distancing [187]. The adjective "physical" is more appropriate than "social" to the word "distancing." Both adjectives have often been used in several grocery and merchandise stores as well as media, although there is a subtle psychological difference. Physical distancing is often much more accepted than mask-wearing because it allows our mind to recognize the individuum in front of us. Nordic, North-European, or Scandinavian people may behave differently from Southern European people. Italians, Greeks, or Spanians living in North Europe love to interconnect a party, or a house invitation is often accompanied by hugging and kissing each other. These populations' acceptance of physical distancing may be critical because they understand a different behavior in living in other countries. The reaction to wearing a mask is variably interpreted. The response is different according to sex/gender, income level, and political affiliation. It has been demonstrated that women are more often able to accept mask-wearing than men. However, both income and political affiliations have been exploited by mass media to appropriate one faction or the other. The income level may not be a decisive factor, but if the individuum is an employee or a self-employeed, the situation may differ. The reason is that being an employee leaves the individuum no or limited choice in accepting any decision coming from the direction or government. At the same time, self-employees feel their freedom is threatened when an entity governs them. Similarly, both conservatives and liberals or socialists have expressed an opinion in favor or against masks, although most anti-maskers seem to belong more to right-wing groups. Said that any political affiliation and mass media polarization in terms of healthy starts on the wrong foot and risks contaminate public health decisions.

The Delphi method is often used in public health, industry, and the economy to reach a mutual agreement [188]. In ancient Greece, the Oracle of Delphi was a place where a priestess located at the temple of Apollo was often asked and well-known for her prophecies. In the Delphi method, individuals allow experts to work toward a mutual agreement by conducting a circulating series of questionnaires and releasing related feedback to discuss each subsequent round further. The ultimate result of the Delphi method is meant to be a true consensus of what the group thinks. One critical persuasion method is portraying agreement. When you show people that a mindset is shared (or not) by others, they are quite keen to adopt it. Witnessing someone wearing a mask makes it more probably that others will do the same. Therefore, persuasion strategies could make sure that people perceive mask-wearing as widespread– perhaps by depicting it frequently in the media or making it compulsory in certain places. We also know from former studies that people are more likely to conform with public health guidelines if they receive clear, precise, consistent, and straightforward procedures. Also, they rely on the source from which they come. But the efficacy of these sorts of "one-size-fits-all" approaches to encouragement and behavioral change are likely to be narrow. Initial findings in the area of personalized influence suggest it might be more effective to try bespoke strategies for people based on combinations of their essential characteristics (their "psychographic profiles") [187]. It seems that three leading personality profiles are critical. Those who are diffident, socially inhibited, and anxious tend to be more likely to be persuaded by those harboring authority. Those who are more self-oriented and calculating tend to feel to be in the opposite corner. These individuals say they are less likely to be influenced by authority figures. The third group i.e., agreeable, extroverted, and conscientious people, report being more likely to be persuaded to do something consistent with what they have done before and less likely if it requires them to change their position. It indicates if they have decided in the past that wearing masks is an awful thing, they are more likely to resist any subsequent efforts to make them wear one or even accept vaccination policies.

Chapter 6

Rage and Scapegoating

Abstract

Rage can quickly destroy humankind and be a stimulus to understand our limits and reformat ourselves. Anger can be induced by xenophobic behaviors and needs to mitigate by cultivating resiliency and prudence. The consideration that rage may have on the psychology of our friends, neighbors, and even ourselves in the long term is crucial. Therefore, having a non-tolerance approach to xenophobia is critical. Xenophobia may let slide our rational approach to scapegoating because it is this procedure the most effortless approach to solve issues, but scapegoating may have dreadful consequences for our society. Thus, stability is paramount to make wise decisions.

Keywords: blaming, rage, scapegoating, society, tolerance

Cosmopolis is the labeling given to a city inhabited by individuals coming from different parts of the world. Considering the grandiosity of the Roman and British Empires and the United States of America, most probably, ancient Rome, London of Great Britain, and New York from the USA are three examples of cities that may be considered harboring and nourishing a cosmopolitan culture. Cosmopolitan areas are beneficial to understand different cultures, and children growing up in a multiethnic environment are keener to influence political and social decisions globally. However, events may trigger rage and scapegoats, and the current pandemic is just one of the numerous examples encountered in history. Since the beginning, cosmopolitan cities are not devoid of intolerance phenomenons, and rage has been a leitmotiv during this pandemic. Rage is defined as violent, cruel, and uncontrolled anger associated with intense feelings perpetrated by a not insane individual. Rage can be factual but also fictitious. Rage is often verbal, and the words we use may trigger violent reactions. The frustration cantered the waves of souls, and political elections at provincial or national levels have been disrupted in multiple countries. A status of imbalance in the soul may drive rage, which may move consequent political decisions in directions, which can be quite different in a balanced soul.

Rage control will be critical in the 21st century. Rage is the opposite of calmness, contentment, serenity, and tranquillity. Nevertheless, rage may positively affect inciting revolts against injustice or crimes, but needs to be short, nonpersonal, and elicits final positive actions. The Control Master Theory is a technique used by therapists [189]. This cognitive, interpersonal, psychoanalytic approach aims to classify behavior as either growth-promoting or pathogenic. In psychoanalysis, this technique is designed to break the blame/rage cycle. However, alternative methods to break the blame/rage cycle and limit the exterior noise are crucial. Climate change activists have invigorated the actions of several countries to fight an inevitable increase in carbon dioxide emissions in the world. However, a trend in rage and destruction of climate change activists may have counterproductive effects. It is easy to be intolerant of leaders that may show their temper. Fingerpointing some leaders just because their reaction is not what we wish may not be the most appropriate approach. At the moment, we finger point, we use a tactic to deliver a product fated ultimately to fail. The blame/rage cycle continues without interruption. Mass media will benefit eventually. Constructive criticisms are crucial and may be delivered using appropriate channels. Feeling angry is a natural outcome of despair, and it is entirely understandable that angry feelings are present. Still, they can be counterproductive and somewhat destructive if not controlled [190-

193]. Rage can also be triggered in individuals when their words are misinterpreted, and verbicide social media have constantly been present in the last few years. The quest for serenity is a natural approach of the human being as well as other animals. Jean Désy, a Canadian physician and writer at the Université Laval, Quebec City, Quebec, has written an essential book on the Nordic feeling [194]. The importance of custody of the words and venerating the silence and nature is critical for nearing the Divine (*Ai-je la foi? Oui, quand je m'intègre à une Nature emportée qui me laisse toute la place nécessaire pour rêver, dans une forêt d'automne, entre les hêtres jaunes et les érables rouges, ou dans la toundra, au cœur de l'immense désert vivant du Grand Nord. Alors, Dieu se manifeste. Je l'entends, sans rien entendre, je le sens dans le silence, ce Dieu qui se trouve entre mes oreilles comme au plus intime de mon ventre* [Do i have faith? Yes, when I integrate myself into a Nature that leaves me the necessary room to dream, in an autumn forest, between yellow beeches and red maples, or in the tundra, in the heart of the immense living desert of the Far North. So, God manifests himself. I hear him, without hearing anything, I feel him in the silence, this God who is between my ears as in the most intimate of my viscera]) [194]. The importance of the minimalism supported by Jean Désy cannot be better laid out with his magnificent words.

Blaming can be active or passive. It is an intrinsic aspect of human beings to reallocate responsibilities onto others, identify a culprit, find a victim or scapegoat and determine a target [195]. During this COVID-19 pandemic, we saw a war of words between the USA, China, and other countries. Not consistently, SARS-CoV-2 was called "Chinese or China virus" or, even more specifically, "Wuhan virus," or sarcastic words such as "Kung-Flu" and "CCP" viruses for the Chinese Communist Party. These words have been repeatedly transmitted on social media [196]. All these words have political and xenophobic implications. Rage may indeed disturb our soul and, it is understandable that the enormous progress reached through a slow economic recovery went jeopardized by a virus. Still, the custody of the words is necessary and prudent. In the past, the Chinese communities experienced multiple episodes of racism, such as in the San Francisco area of the last century. The sufferance of these Chinese

Americans in previous epidemics should let us reflect before words are pronounced that may harbor a xenophobic connotation. The internment of American and Canadian Japanese and Italian people during WWII has been atrocious. A 38-year long head tax was levied against Chinese immigrants starting in 1885. These acts and other structural impediments infringed upon human rights.

Our body is a temple, as Paul, the apostle, mentions in his epistle to Corinthians. Our body is to glorify God (*An nescitis quoniam membra vestra, templum sunt Spiritus Sancti, qui in vobis est, quem habetis a Deo, et non estis vestri? Empti enim estis pretio magno. Glorificate, et portate Deum in corpore vestro*) ["You do not know that your body is a temple of the Holy Ghost which is in you, which you have from God, and you are not your own? Since you are priceless, glorify and keep God in your body"] [197]. We are in charge of what our mouth expresses, and caution should be exercised to avoid injury and damage to our citizen fellows. The Chinese Americans share the same country and often the same citizenship and roots of suffering similar to many other communities. The idea that Americans with European heritage are more Americans than Americans coming from other countries is evil. There is no part of the Canadian Chart of Rights, Declaration of the Independence, or Constitution of the United States of America indicating it. All people are equal, and all lives matter, no matter the skin color or ethnic background. During this pandemic and before, negative racial attitudes and racial bias have increased worldwide, mainly when xenophobic views are expressed and accepted. This behavior has a considerable physical, mental, social, and economic burden with prolonged effects on the well-being of the countries [198, 199]. The community-level racial climate is related to cardiovascular outcomes, mortality, and even birth outcomes [200-205]. There is a pseudo-doctrine of an ideology exhibiting racial inferiority in the larger society's values, language, imagery, symbols, and unstated assumptions in cultural racism. Media, stereotyping, fashion, behavior are inside of cultural racism. Cultural racism is systemic by producing a toxic environment where individuals live when racism resides, let alone institutional and individual-level discrimination at all levels. Such attitudes have been intrinsically associated with both mental and physical health outcomes [206].

Internet is a great resource for education and entrainment, and its proliferation has resulted in an astonishingly growing number of online social networks and discussion forums in the last decade. Commonly, most social media enforce a real-name policy. In contrast, some media have the opportunity to leave users anonymous, supporting some privacy advocates who claim that real-name policies would erode online freedom [207]. Twitter, a social media platform, allows users to keep anonymous. The absence of a real-name policy supported the expansion of Twitter as a popular exchange gateway for consumers to share and access information without being detectable [208, 209]. The anonymity perceived or real of such social media will inevitably decrease the self-control or power or internal censorship for socially unacceptable views. This behavior increases the inclination to express less likely reported attitudes in survey interviews due to social desirability bias [210]. Studies aiming to describe difference in racial feeling based on the sentiment of tweets using race-related terms before and following the rise of COVID-19 is far to be perfect but may indicate a disgregation of the society. Nguyen et al. utilized an Application Programming Interface (API) on Twitter's Streaming to collect more than three millions US race-related tweets from November 2019–June 2020 [198]. A supervised machine learning model labeled support vector machine (SVM) was used to study the sentiment analysis. Although these studies on social media have been subjected to controversial approval and judgments, there is some accuracy. It was estimated that such precision for identifying negative sentiments, comparing the machine learning model to manually labeled tweets, was 91% raising data that can be analyzed on sociology and public health levels. The authors studied changes in racial sentiment before and following the rise of the COVID-19 pandemic. They found that the proportion of negative tweets referencing Asians increased by 68.4%. It has been reported an increase from 9.8% in November 2019 (USA-China trade war) to about 16.5% in March 2020. Some common themes surfaced during the content analysis, including blame and racism (20%), anti-racism (20%), but daily life impact themes were slightly more dominant (27%). The rate of negative tweets referencing other racial/ethnic minorities remained relatively stable during this period. Xenophobic internet searches spiked in late January 2020. The World Health Organization (WHO) correctly and, in a tempestive manner, released guidelines in February 2020 advising against the use of stigmatizing language about COVID-19 [211].

Tweets, newspaper articles, and interviews continue using national labeling. Also, German measles, Spanish Flu, or Middle East Respiratory Syndrome (another Coronavirus) are often terms used in scientific papers. Nevertheless, labeling as a "Chinese virus" is inappropriate in this context because it can incite and escalate racist sentiments. These sentiments continue to be quite high during the fight between conservative-republican and democratic-liberal parties. The USA-China trade war never satisfactorily ended, but a note is that probably more than 90% of the products sold are manufactured in China. Disgracefully, a rise in anti-Asian hate crimes was documented and culminated in the tragic Atlanta shooting [212]. However, anti-American messages appeared in the early pandemic in China, supporting conspiracy theories that prolonged well after the pandemic was under control in China. The Chinese data are difficult to collect and analyzed because the CCP heavily monitors WeChat. The innocuous social dimension of WeChat has been perverted. Such technology became a powerful weapon in tightening censorship. The state controls the citizens both in the mainland and overseas [213]. There is no more American or less American or more Canadian or less Canadian because all live in the same world. Disrespect or racism should not be tolerated in academia, industry, or any other environment [38]. Diversity and multiculturalism are the strength of a nation, and numerous Chinese Americans or Americans with Chinese origin are heavily critics of the CCP or Chinese government. Still, they do not or cannot express their feelings or evaluations because they are afraid for the relatives living in China that may be the subject of attacks. Remarkably, negative racist sentiments and anti-American or Anti-Chinese feelings existed before the COVID-19 pandemic. In the United States, it was generally higher for other racial and ethnic groups (e.g., African Americans and Latinx) than Asians. On the other side of the ocean and vehemently, both Chinese official politicians and media exacerbated the blame game.

Chinese officials launched a defamatory campaign hitting the ball back to the US, trying to shift the blame. A Chinese official, the Foreign Ministry spokesman Lijian Zhao, wrote, "It might be (the) US army who brought the epidemic to Wuhan. Be transparent! Make public your data! US owe us an explanation!" [214]. Also, People's Daily, the largest newspaper group in China and the official newspaper of the Central Committee of the CCP, publishing worldwide with a circulation of 3 million, published on March 19th, 2020 an article with the title "Don't fall for it! Trump is using 'Chinese virus' label to cover up his mishandling of Coronavirus" [196]. Supported by anti-Western nationalism, the US was often labeled the "Enemy of the world" [215, 216]. In addition to blaming the USA for spreading COVID-19, Chinese officials have started to trigger a movement on Chinese social media to disentangle China from the negative COVID-19 narrative and proposing the CCP as a compassionate corporation that unselfishly helps others, especially strangers. This narrative emphasizing the Good Samaritan policy and providing medical assistance and PPE to numerous countries is key in influencing both people and foreign governments. This narrative did not occur, however, without benefit either of an image or economically. Outrageously, blaming is an insidious process.

Blame games are universal and not only limited between the USA and China. In Italy, the Southern provinces blamed some Northern Italians who originally migrated from the South to travel back to the South and bring the Northern virus into the South. The same situation happened in Quebecers returning from Spain and Italy. Southern European member states accused the European Union (EU) of being too slow in helping the member states questioning the validity of Europe. Jewish communities around the globe reported an increase in anti-Semitic incidents during the pandemic, like the Medieval Age pandemic. India had also experienced acts of racism when Muslims were blamed for the spread of the virus [217]. Paranoic sinophobia increased exponentially. Similarly, anti-Western sentiments among Chinese communities have been registered all over the world. Numerous mixed marriages have been jeopardized even broken if an immediate action to mitigate media damage and emphasize family value was not undertaken. The LGBTQ community, which involves individuals with lesbian, gay, bisexual, and transgender behavior, has been the target of attacks from both media and government authorities in South Korea and other countries, similar to what happened for the Human Immunodeficiency Virus pandemic a few decades ago [217]. The backlash against the LGBTQ community is insane because of the historical discrimination against this community crossing borders and countries. In Turkey, the top Muslim cleric Ali Erbas triggered open indignation worldwide when he indicated that same-sex relations were responsible for the pandemic marking the first day of Ramadan [218].

Hypocrisy may accompany blaming. The Ebola virus represents a moral challenge for our world on both an individual and collective level [219]. In China, the risk of an Ebola Virus Disease (EVD) pandemic created a justified atmosphere of fear in public because of frequent trade activities between China and African countries. Guangzhou is the capital and most crowded city of the province of Guangdong in southern China. This city is an important international trading hub and home to more than 20,000 African residents [220]. Bodomo's analysis suggests that the number of African migrants in Guangzhou could easily be more than 100,000 as the Republic Popular of China is the leading trade partner with Africa. It has also been suggested that an average of 2.8 infected travelers a month would be departing from the three EVD-affected countries (Guinea, Liberia, and Sierra Leone) if no appropriate exit screening measures were put in place [221]. According to the WHO's Ebola dashboard [222], the Democratic Republic of the Congo (DRC) identified five more Ebola cases at the beginning of January 2021. On February 7th, 2021, the DRC Minister declared an outbreak of EVD after the laboratory confirmation of one case in North Kivu Province [223]. Since Guangzhou is one of the top 25 final destinations for flights from these countries, it is realistic to assume that Guangzhou may have been under the threat of an Ebola outbreak at any time. During the Ebola outbreak, which occurred a few years ago, the China Health Department implemented a temperature monitoring system to reinforce the surveillance of travelers. Moreover, an unofficial quarantine of recent African travelers from the Ebola-affected countries (Guinea, Libera, Sierra Leone, and DRC) was imposed in Guangzhou [224]. The prevention measures were of exceptional high level, including body temperature twice daily and quarantine for 21 days carrying a Global Positioning System (GPS)-enabled mobile phone at all times. These measures were apparently selected only for Black Africans. At the same time, little has been commented about the effort to monitor the more than 1,000 Chinese medical workers, investors, and other foreigners who have traveled to the affected countries since the outbreak began. It has been argued that prevention efforts were applied universally to people at risk for carrying the infection, but a Lancet article goes in a different direction. In China, racial discrimination is a major concern among African migrants and has been brought to social platforms as a form of hypocrisy [225]. It is important to remember that carrying foreign status is already a barrier to access health information and services [226]. Dirlikov and Jiang sustain that as a result of EVD-related stigma, the African migrants became more susceptible to discrimination [227]. Also, educating the public about the virus and its spread may reduce racial discrimination and stigma against African migrants living in China and other countries [228]. A similar situation occurred for the COVID-19 pandemic. Most of the media have poorly treated these aspects because they were very much interested in blaming the former President of the United States and the Republican Party for anti-Chinese comments. According to Human Rights Watch, discriminatory treatment in China against Africans is still present despite the "zero-tolerance" policy against racism of the government. Africans and people of African origin experience discrimination in employment, accommodation, and other domains. In Guangzhou, a campaign started in early April 2020 to forcibly test Africans for SARS-CoV-2, ordering them to self-isolate or confine in designated hotels. This treatment was not initially reserved for non-Black people entering China. There have been numerous examples of landlords evicting African residents, obliging many to sleep on the street or assigned hotels, apparently, at their costs. Also, shops and restaurants refused African customers for fear that some individuals harbored the virus [229]. Even if some news may have been amplified because officials in China are not allowed to talk to foreign journalists, it is of major concern that Africans feel that way after allowing Chinese companies affiliated with the CCP to build infrastructures in Africa trading for natural resources. Actions targeting

Africans and African Americans, allegedly in the name of disease control, have shaken the foreign student community in Guangzhou, a city with extraordinary academic excellence [230]. Several disturbing reports were circulating on social media, and some resentment against some Africans is common. Racism may still be a ‘barrier’ for African students in China despite a florid and prosperous bilateral and economic relationship. Although the Chinese government, which has used generous scholarships and other programs to attract more than 80,000 African students to the country, acted quickly, racism and discrimination will persist [231]. A TV commercial advert for a Chinese laundry detergent has been widely condemned, with comments pointing out that it is the most racist commercial ever to be screened. However, this is very similar to one made by Italians in Italy [232]. A young black man winks and whistles at a Chinese girl, who flirtatiously beckons him towards her, before putting a pouch of liquid detergent in his mouth and pushing him head-first into the washing machine. At the end of the washing cycle, the man who emerges is a fair-skinned man. On the other hand, a black journalist ‘SNL’s Michael Che, NBC, has been accused of ‘antisemitic trope’ in the ‘Weekend Update’ segment for anti-Semitism accusing Israel of a “joke” of vaccinating only Jews. Every Israeli, including Jew, Muslim, Christian, or other religious groups, was eligible for the COVID jab. He had to retract and apologize [233]. Migrants and refugees are at risk for blaming and health issues. We recently pointed out how migrants and refugees are at higher risk of osteoporosis and other complications other than mental health issues. These aspects need to be targeted in programs aimed at annihilating racism in our society [234]. The partiality of some news outlets is particularly overwhelming considering the enormous polarization of several academic institutions against either conservatives or free speech. In reality, no race or ethnics is immune against the evil of racism, which can be very subtle, pervasive, and unjustified. Even if governments support zero-tolerance policies against racism, it is present worldwide and can have several degrees and nuances.

Racism is a complex phenomenon that needs to be not only discouraged but also debellated. The problem of racism has been targeted only on one side, but it may need to be considered a form of *mis*-dialogue. Dialogue is a critical word indicating the opportunity to communicate between at least two entities or two individuals using a way of communication. Dialogue comes from Late Latin "*Dialogus*," which arises from the Ancient Greek word διάλογος "conversation, discourse," which is a combination of διά "through, inter" and λόγος "speech," διαλέγομαι, and λέγειν "to speak." Thus, a dialogue occurs when the speech or discourse occurs using a kind of bridge or communication tool and the two or more entities speak and listen to each other alternatively. It may be considered a locus or space of equality and civility in which the two parts which may differ may speak and listen alternatively. The centrality of the word dialogue is in the prefix διά, which is crucial. It makes the word different from monologue or soliloquy, which is a speech presented by a single character in a drama or a theatrical event. In the monologue, which derives from the Byzantine Greek μονόλογος "speaking alone," there is only one entity or individual often expressing thoughts aloud, with or without rhetorically addressing any other entity or individual from the audience. Monologues or soliloquies are not communicating or building bridges. The late Latin word *sōliloquium* is in St. Augustine's work entitled *Soliloquiorum Libri duo* or Two Books of Soliloquies [235]. In dialogue, it has been suggested that we seek to put aside fears, angst, or the need to win. In the dialogue, there is a willingness to listen to other options or voices. The implementation of dialogue supports the opportunity to work out tensions, paradoxes, and even preconceptions. Diana Chapman Walsh was President of Wellesley College from 1993 to 2007. During her tenure, the college revised its curriculum and expanded its programs in global education, internships and service-learning, and interdisciplinary teaching and learning. Diana Chapman Walsh describes the dialogue this way "It's when we let our guard down and allow our differences and doubts to surface and interact that something authentic and original can begin to emerge, tentatively, in the spaces between us. And I've found that it's often in these fleeting and complicated moments that the heart and mind can come into synchrony, pointing to altogether novel educational possibilities. The key is to remain alert to those moments and to move with them when they arise. We know that the most effective process for discovering these layers of meaning is through interactive and iterative dialogues. If we undertake them sincerely and openly—and patiently—we can sometimes find our way to something entirely new. We assume that individual voices speak and act for the system as a whole. We listen carefully or a variety of voices and the competing values they represent" [236]. Also, Al-Gore specifies, "...it is now connection that is the key. A well-connected community is made up of men and women who discuss and debate ideas and issues among themselves. They constantly test the validity of the information and impressions they receive from one another—as well as the ones they receive from their government" [236]. Racism is a *mis-dialogue*, not a monologue. It is the inefficient and ineffective communication between two individuals or two parties. The *mis*- prefix inoculates the word hate in the community. The word μισέω arises from the Greek and means "I hate." It is crucial in understanding this concept. Racism is an abnormity involving both parts. Both parts are guilty of the lack of dialogue. It is a very subtle concept but is comparable and assimilable to envy, which is the longing or desire to possess a quality, an attribute, or an object belonging to someone else. Cicero was a Roman statesman, lawyer, and scholar who played an important role in the politics of the Roman Republic, upholding optimate principles during several political crises. Cicero indicates that "*invidia non in eo qui invidet solum dicitur, sed etiam in eo cui invidetur*," i.e., therefore it is said to be envy not only who is envious, but also in that to which it is envied (Cic. Tusc. 3, 9, 20) [29]. This sentence is a critical concept inserted in the *Tusculanae Disputationes* emphasizing minimalism and frugality, two qualities that are characteristic aspects of stoicism against any form of racism.

Assimilation is the absorption and digestion of nutrients or food by the body or any specific biological system. Also, it regards the process of taking in and fully understanding information or ideas. In cultural assimilation, a minority group or culture resembles a society's majority group or assumes the values, behaviors, and beliefs of another group [38]. Unfortunately, it has received a negative connotation, but it may harbor positive and negative aspects with fruitful products if fears and preconceptions are solved. Phobia is a kind of anxiety disorder characterized by a persistent and, probably, excessive apprehension or fear of an object or situation. One of the most common phobias known in both children and adults, is arachnophobia, i.e., anxiety or reaction to spiders. While social phobia is an anxiety disorder in which the individual experiences a dreadful situation as the person is worried about other peers judging him or her, xenophobia is the fear or dislike of foreigners, aliens, or visitors the unknown individuals. Xenophobia, which derives from the Greek ξένος "stranger" or "foreigner" and φόβος "fear," is often used to describe or label nationalistic political beliefs and movements. In 2019, a survey conducted by the Pew Research Center indicated that 76% of Black and Asian respondents had suffered some form of intolerance [237]. Xenophobia, as indicated before, is not a current phenomenon involving the United States and Canada only. Almost all countries and ethnicities have experienced or expressed some xenophobic views of variable degrees. Xenophobia was even present in the Ancient World. It is commonly seen in texts the consideration of the Greek culture as upper class. The Greeks denigrated aliens as "barbarians" with a strong belief that the Greek culture was superior to any other known world culture. Ancient Romans were less opened to express xenophobic views because, for the Roman culture, citizenship involved privileges and duties. The most important aspect was that everybody had to pay taxes to Rome no matter which region was taken early or late during the Roman empire's expansion. Thus, one of the primary reasons for the destruction of the Jerusalem temple was the impossibility of receiving taxes from Jews. There are, however, examples of speeches regarded as xenophobic in Ancient Roman history. Christians were, however, considered of a lower level and targeted as individuals to extinguish. Xenophobic discourses, although rare, were also present in Ancient Rome. There was some xenophobia against Macedonians, Thracians, Illyrians, and Syrians [238]. The Harvard entomologist Edward O. Wilson claimed that xenophobia is universal. It may have a genetic basis [239]. The "Dawkins" selfish gene hypothesis argued that the unit of evolutionary selection must be an active, germ-line replicator [240]. It is difficult to prove in detail these theories, but, interestingly, the biology of fear- and anxiety-related behaviors has been under intense neuroscientific investigation [241].

Xenophobia and anxiety may also have a relatively well-established physiological substrate, and the connection between psychology and neurochemistry may be a topic of investigation in the nearest future. In a state of fear or anxiety, autonomic activation and increased arousal as early physiological and psychological responses have been identified. The *locus coeruleus*, an area of the brain localized in the pons of the brainstem, is involved with physiological responses to stress and panic. It seems that such areas are the core around which feelings of anxiety are arranged. Interestingly, the *locus ceruleus* contains many cells harboring noradrenaline cell bodies and is considered the critical region involved in arousal. In vertebrates, like monkeys, rats, and cats, an increased neuronal firing rate is associated with alertness, vigilance, and selective attention to meaningful and/or novel stimuli. The vulnerability to anxiety seems to be generated by an abnormal balance between the activity of the septo-hippocampal behavioral inhibition system (BIS), the behavioral approach system (BAS), and the fight/flight system (F/FLS). Also, three specific sites in the brain are associated with a complete fear response, including the central and lateral zones of the amygdala, the anterior and medial hypothalamus, and well-determined areas of the periaqueductal gray (PAG). LeDoux et al. studied a simple fear conditioning paradigm in rats and identified that the amygdala plays a primary role in controlling emotional and social behaviors. Bilateral lesions of the amygdala in adult macaque monkeys provoke a lack of fear response to inanimate objects. Also, a "socially uninhibited" behavioral pattern has been recorded. It seems that an amygdala dysregulation or imbalance may be at the basis of social anxiety. Moreover, specific phobias may originate in the basolateral nucleus of the amygdala [241].

The risk of scapegoating minorities is to create a world of inferior versus superior individuals. "*Scapegoating is the practice of singling out any party for unmerited negative treatment or blame. Although, in many cases, the scapegoat is an individual (whether a child, employee, or peer), there are plenty of examples of ethnic or religious groups, divisions of a business, government departments, industry sectors, and even whole countries*" according to Dr. Graham Wilson [242]. As reported by Tacitus, in the

Annals, on July 64 AD, Rome was devastated by a great fire that lasted for nine days [243]. The fire was monstrous in that it destroyed a large part of the city, including the imperial palace on the Palatine. Nero was the fifth Roman emperor, ruling from 54 to 68 AD. He somewhat managed Roman society in the first ten years of government, although a hostile environment diffused quickly. In these areas, the idea or conspiracy that the emperor was the author himself to cause fire spread like an oil stain on water. The idea was that the Emperor caused the fire because he was eager to modernize the city and to embellish it with new buildings, but there is no safe proof that he was the culprit of the fire despite controversial issues. He was in Anzio (51 kilometers/32 miles south of Rome) when the fire broke out, and most of his most precious treasures were destroyed due to the fire. Nero was exceedingly jealous about his treasure and there is no proof that he was affected with masochistic personality disorder. Nevertheless, Pliny the Elder, Suetonius, and some other anti-imperial historians wrote that Nero was responsible for the Great Fire of Rome. After evaluating data, Tacitus, an impartial Roman historiographic and historian and, probably, the primary ancient source for information about the fire, reported ineluctably that the fire was an accident. Yet, Nero remains famous for Rome's fire. Nero rushed to Rome promptly, worked incessantly to extinguish the fire, and started immediate support and reconstruction. Nero favored the homeless and the injured Romans, but despite all the great works he profused, he could not remove the vile accusation of arsonist spreading against and around him. The hostility rose, and his worries to keep the empire united were devised to find a scapegoat in the Christians. The community believers were considered subverters of the typical social order. Most of the people assumed that Christians were practicing rites that were deemed blasphemous. After summary trials, the Christians were accused and kept responsible for the Great Fire of Rome. Spectacles of cruelty with people beaten and burned alive proliferate with a revolutionary ferocity against individuals harboring the Christian life [243]. As indicated in Leviticus, the third book of the Torah and the Old Testament, Aaron, a high priest and the elder brother of Moses shall cast lots upon the two goats.Substantially, one lot for the Lord, and the other lot for Azazel (16:8 לרוגו הוהיל דחא לרוג תולרג םריעשה ינש לע ןרהא ןתנו

dna ,droL eht rof llef tol eht hcihw nopu taog eht tneserp llahs ,(אחד לעזאזל offer him for a sin-offering (16:9 לרוגה וילע הלע רשא ריעשה תא ןרהא בירקהו tes eb llahs ,lezazA rof llef tol eht hcihw no ,taog eht dna ,(ליהוה ועשהו חטאת alive before the Lord, to make atonement over him, to send him away for Azazel into the wilderness (16:10 ינפל יח דמעי לזאזעל לרוגה וילע הלע רשא ריעשהו (המדברה לעזאזל אתו לשלח עליו לכפר יהוה[244]. Thus, of the pair, one goat was sacrificed (not the "scapegoat"), while the other goat (the "scapegoat") was released into the wilderness, taking with it all sins. There is antonomasia for the Hebraic tradition of the Day of Atonement. The pure are the victims, while the culprits are the scapegoat causing or taking the sins and impurities. Scapegoating is the process by which a person or individuals are blamed for something that they did not do. The actual origin of the problem is either never identified or purposely ignored, as displayed in textbooks of social psychology and psychiatry [195]. Blaming and scapegoating are associated with rage. Scapegoating often occurs when individuals suffer without the definite possibility of fighting, evidence of psychological or physical distress, or experiencing significant damage or oppression. These blame games can become vicious and run in a vicious circle. Of course, rationality may well help to discern this process, but anger, hate, and resentment often obscure it [195]. Lozano & Laurent (2019) pointed out that we live in a culture where people are strongly motivated to avoid responsibility. In this current culture, people do not want to appear blameworthy and are ready to point their fingers at anyone but themselves when things go wrong [245].

Blaming and scapegoating are easy picks. In 2021, a year after the pandemic started, blaming continues through a systematic disinformation campaign on both Chinese and non-Chinese social media. Although the WHO has downplayed a Chinese theory that SARS-CoV-2 was brought to Wuhan through frozen food, some conspiracy theories surfaced on the internet. Two investigators, Vladimir Dedkov from the Pasteur Institute in St Petersburg, Russia, and Fabian Leendertz, an emerging diseases specialist at Robert Koch Institute, Berlin, Germany, had an interview with the Financial Times. They indicated that it was improbable the first cases of SARS-CoV-2 identified in Wuhan in 2019 entered the city on frozen or refrigerated goods because there were no widespread outbreaks of COVID-

19 in food factories around the world [246]. Another conspiracy theory suggests that the virus was brought to Wuhan by a delegation of US athletes during an international competition. These narratives underline the highly charged geopolitics surrounding the roots of COVID-19 [246]. It is unlikely that the COVID-19 origin will be adequately investigated because of the initial coverups and late investigations. In this setting, it is unavoidable that conspiracy theories and fake news have essentially invaded the internet weakening our rationale [247]. Another conspiracy theory points out a virology lab leaking. The laboratory leak theory is presented in a pre-print manuscript, but numerous flaws are present in this manuscript. Dr. Gkikas Magiorkinis, Assistant Professor of Hygiene and Epidemiology and Scientific Coordinator of the National Reference Centre for Retroviruses, National and Kapodistrian University of Athens, analyzed the SARS-CoV-2 genome. The Public Health expert compared SARS-CoV-2 with the sequences of other coronaviruses by molecular evolution analyses. The genome of SARS-CoV-2 is more than 95% like another coronavirus, RaTG13, isolated from bats. In another study, SARS-CoV-2-related coronaviruses were identified in Malayan pangolins suggesting that such animals are animal reservoirs [248]. The retrieval of closely related coronaviruses from animals such as bats and pangolins makes the scenario of naturally occurring evolution far more likely than any scenario of laboratory manipulation. The pre-print does not provide any robust evidence of artificial manipulation and no statistical test of alternative hypotheses [249]. Dr. Daniel Altmann, Professor of Immunology, Imperial College London, indicates that most of the bulk of data supports bats or pangolins' origins [247]. Such speculations may damage public health efforts to keep COVID-19 cases low [250]. Also, the spike glycoprotein of SARS-CoV-2 contains a potential cleavage site for furin proteases, which are highly biologically active proteins able to process latent precursor proteins into their biologically active products. The furin recognition motif present at the SARS-CoV-2 S1/S2 junction has no analogy in other "linage B" β-CoVs, including neither pangolin-CoV nor RaTG13, suggesting that the S protein S1/S2 junction is not a hot spot for RNA recombination termination highlighting the improbability of artificial virus technology [251].

Peer review and honesty are fundamental in science and academia. There is danger coming from propagating not robust data as accurate. We may recall the 1998 Wakefield et al.'s paper stating that the vaccine against measles, mumps, and rubella (MMR vaccine) may lead to autism spectrum disorders [252]. Wakefield and coauthors reported 12 children with ileal lymphoid nodular hyperplasia, non-specific colitis, and neuropsychological symptoms. In this manuscript, the authors hypothesized that the MMR vaccine could trigger bowel dysfunction leading to gastrointestinal absorption of neurotoxic peptides. There would be resulting damage to the central nervous system, and autism spectrum disorders can occur. Although the hypothesis was scientifically stimulating, this manuscript was found to be fraudulent. However, it was retracted 12 years later. Both ethical and misconduct committees investigated the data of this paper and found noticeable missing results. Thus, the hypothesis was not adequately investigated, raising concerns about the quality of the peer reviewers of a high impact factor journal. The disaster is that the retraction occurred 12 years later, the online publication [253]. It means that it triggered conspiracy theories and divulgated parental concerns about the safety of the MMR vaccine, ultimately leading to lower vaccination levels and outbreaks of measles infection in several countries. An evidence-based meta-analysis of five cohort studies with more than one million patients and five case-control studies with about ten thousand patients found no evidence for a link between MMR vaccination and the subsequent development of autism or autistic spectrum disorders [254]. Humanity is on edge not due to COVID-19 but because honesty and transparency may often be missing. Thus, we need to go back to the proper reasoning of any scientific process before supporting conspiracy theories.

Narrative change around COVID-19 is a key factor in the Chinese leadership and has been a topic of intense acrimony. Raj Verma is the Head of Research at Huaqiao University, Guangzhou, China. Dr. Verma analyzed these events scrupulously from a social-political perspective. He suggested three reasons why Chinese officials are trying to change the narrative regarding the current COVID-19 pandemic [215, 216]. China has an eager quest for great power status. The trillion-dollar Belt and Road Initiative, accompanied by multilateral financial institutions, such as the Silk Road Fund and the Asian Infrastructure Investment Bank, are examples of this strategy. In more than 100 countries, China became a key component of globalization with an incalculable number of factories in the country. China provides financial assistance, loans, and building infrastructure worldwide. However, this assistance comes with the scrutiny of the laws and behavior of these countries in the international relationship. Substantially, most financial assistance and loans presuppose loyalty and respect for China's countries at the national and international levels. The subjugation of several sports leagues and universities is blatant and has been exposed on several platforms. The Chinese leadership may have important issues in the global perceptions regarding Chinese trade. The virus outbreak may let the world focus on China's intrusive government, but the costly private healthcare system is not secondary. The initial failed response to the virus outbreak, which has been astutely cleared off in Chinese social media, is appalling. In the first few months, Chinese citizens exchanged several messages on WeChat and other Chinese social media about a new virus outbreak. These messages are dissipated, and the few officials have been removed from their position and displaced to other peripheral provinces. The Chinese leadership or CCP is afraid that Chinese citizens may highlight some local shortcomings of its political system. Since most of the population has not been exposed to the strengths and weaknesses of Western democracies, students returning to China may have good jobs, which provide a good income and family support. These students are reluctant to attack their leadership because they may jeopardize their status. This behavior is perfectly human, logical, and comprehensible. The Chinese leadership is also concerned that the developed world might blame China for the global recession. This blame is particularly worrying to the leadership because it would sound like a mortal knell for China's reputation. The consequence could be a devastating shift of manufacturing and trade away from Chinese territories. In the past, Chinese propaganda targeted the United States as an imperial power during the Cold War galvanizing the Chinese public in times of crisis. Public officials working in government posts and most scientists have had their passports controlled or seized under the current presidentship, a phenomenon that never happened with any other Chinese president. The presidency was changed from time-restrained to perennial, which may be unimaginable for Western democracies. Chinese people are indeed poorly informed, and censorship is galoping. The Chinese portray of itself as a Good Samaritan is tremendous. The best manufacturing powerhouse produced and shipped medical equipment such as masks, gloves, and ventilators worldwide. However, some facts are missing. Not only did the United Nations International Children's Emergency Fund donated disinfectants, gloves, protective suits, and face masks to China in the early stage of the pandemic, but the "Enemy of the World" pledged to spend US$100 million to help China and other countries to combat SARS-CoV-2 on the beginning of the pandemic. The United States sent 17.8 tons of medical equipment to China. Also, private companies of the United States donated hundreds of millions of dollars to China. The European Union sent more than 50 tons of medical supplies to China, and the Japanese government and private sector sent medical supplies and made monetary contributions to China. These facts have not been emphasized in the Chinese social platforms because they could jeopardize the politics of discreditation. Chinese citizens were shocked in front of Dr. Li Wenliang's death. It led to an outpouring of national criticism, grief, anger, and mistrust against the CPC, despite being finally declared a national hero. Dr. Li's death became the top trending subject on Chinese social media with an estimated 1.5 billion views. Initially, WeChat and other social platforms were submerged by a multitude of messages inspiring more freedom of speech, demands for the Wuhan government to take concrete action on the subordinate individuals, and calls for a law to protect whistleblowers. All these hashtags have been censored and removed quickly in WeChat. However, some discordant views are inside the CPC, and this may regard far more the initial handling of SARS-CoV-2. An open letter circulated on WeChat. The letter was calling for an emergency meeting of the politburo to discuss some presidential issues. Intergenerational discontents seem to be present in the CPC, and some citizens feel that the current president is behaving like an emperor. Some believe it to be considered the re-incarnation of Mao Zedong. The letter emerged after the disappearance of Ren Zhiqiang, a social media star and property tycoon who criticized the government's response to COVID-19 [216]. Finally, the appetite for expansion of the Chinese leadership is growing. Worrying are the escalations between China and Taiwan. Taiwan is a sovereign country but is considered a renegade province from mainland China. One of the significant efforts and acts of tolerance of Mao Zedong was leaving the Nationalists to withdraw to the island and live there in peace. The re-exacerbation of these contrasts with some acts against Hong Kong dissent and violence is quite disturbing. The danger of a potential *casus belli* like the Gleiwitz incident needs to be taken into account in the future.

Politics is interfering with every aspect of COVID-19, unfortunately, because it is a virus that has a fundamentally tremendous geopolitical influence. The origins, the blocking of whistleblowers, the concealing of some data, the disastrous and ambiguous initial statements of public health officials on face masking and travel bans, the education disruption, the lockdown-related mental issues, the economic damage have been catastrophic. It is genuine to simply shrug and say, 'let's hope for better info someday.' It is an insult to reason and intelligence. Misinterpretations, fake news, conspiracy theories, and political polarization fuel blame games and hostility [255]. It remains the heroism of numerous unknown or less known whistle-blowers like Dr. Li Wenliang, who put their careers and lives on the risk line to alert the public [128, 256]. Heroism, empathy, and altruism are in solid need no matter the country or the ethnicity. We now can rebuild our society compassionately and equitably. Heroism is the natural remedy against the "*homo homini lupus*" (man is wolf to man). Health disparities are present worldwide but also complex both in nature and geographically. Health disparities cannot be easily solved with the nationalization of health services. There are numerous dangers in nationalizing healthcare for everybody [257]. The control of physicians' salaries may have a negative effect on some benefits that may not be profitable. The 24/7 access to physicians, which is present in the private sector, may disappear in restricted budgets unless the expenses of the government for healthcare become unreasonable for any private company to get profit. Moreover, the long waiting lists with months or even years may become a reality, such as in

Canada or the United Kingdom. The risk of nationalization of health care may bring unwanted consequences like history tell us. In 1883, the concept of eugenics was advocated by Francis Galton, who also coined the name [258]. Buck v. Bell, 274 US 200 (1927), is a decision of the United States Supreme Court, written by Justice Oliver Wendell Holmes, Jr. [259]. The Supreme Court ruled that a state may permit compulsory sterilization of the unfit (such as the intellectually disabled) "for the protection and health of the state" because it did not violate the due process clause of the Fourteenth Amendment to the United States Constitution. Apart from Nazi Germany, the forced sterilization of some patients was one of the most popular reforms among political progressives. Tragically, sterilization operated against the feeble-minded epileptics, individuals with mental and physical disabilities, and people with tendencies toward alcoholism, drug abuse, crime, and prostitution. Techniques of cloning or gene editing are well established. It is foreseeable that such sterilization may become a reality in the future. The Lynchburg Story reveals that about 70,000 Americans were forcibly sterilized [260]. The Tuskegee syphilis study reveals the medical profession's conspiracy and betrayal of the Hippocratic Oath with several consequences of mistrust of some Black communities [261-267]. The swine flu vaccination failure of the mid-1970s with several dangerous side effects, including the Guillain-Barre Syndrome, a neurologic syndrome with death as a complication in one out of 20 patients, should be considered [268]. In Canada, liberal views increasingly expand medical assistance in dying (MAID), reminiscent of a eugenic process. Bill C-7 proposes a two-tier system for those whose death is reasonably predictable and those who are not. It allows a waiver of the final consent for those whose death is reasonably foreseeable but who may lose the capacity to consent before MAID can be provided [269]. These are only a few examples of disastrous consequences for the nationalization of health care when the medical profession with politics leads the path of citizens. On the other hand, some countries have failed to address the response to the current pandemic adequately. Some hospitals have been reluctant to take patients who cannot afford co-payment for add-ons not covered in insurance schedules, and India and Kenya are two examples. Still, several Association of Southeast Asian

Nations (ASEAN) countries responded promptly and proactively through unilateral and aggressive legislation or dictating limitations on private providers [270].

Discrimination causes and increases poverty and illness. Physicians need to be at the forefront of addressing inequality as a core social determinant of health for patients. As physicians, we need to tackle the exposure to adverse events with proper incident reporting and optimize vocational and educational attainment for all students, no matter their ethics. The Society of Global Health experience, a Section of the American Academy of Pediatrics, has been crucial in tackling specific disasters and catastrophes worldwide [271]. We need to collaborate with politicians in helping solve substantial societal problems that affect patients of all ages, mainly children. It is paramount not to get upset with people or situations. In both cases, the conditions are powerless without our reaction, which is based on Newton law [12]. However, preservation of momentum or energy is the more fundamental idea. Substantially, we do not react but respond. If we do not react, there will not be any power affecting us. In the end, taking responsibility for thoughts, feelings, and actions is crucial. Rage is not the answer, but calm, pause, and reflection are the pathway for an adequate response to everything and everyone, even COVID-19.

Chapter 7

MENTAL HEALTH AND 21ST CENTURY FAMILY CHALLENGES

ABSTRACT

Mental health is one of the significant challenges of our century, and underpinning efforts to fight this emergency is critical for future generations. The 21st-century challenges are not global but involve the individual. This chapter targets the mental health issues involved in the pandemic and the post-traumatic stress disorders that future generations may show.

Keywords: mental health, challenge, anxiety, drugs, opioid, cannabis

"Am I on a suicide watch, ain't I?" asked Michael to Brian. Brian didn't answer but sat on the stairs close to his house and started starring at two clouds touching the sky. "They came multiple times yesterday in my room to look for something," added Michael. "They took away all my pencils and pens and all plastic bags," starring the sky again. I came across this nonfictional adolescent narrative a few times during this pandemic. It is only a sign that mental health youth is rapidly declining, and all of us may be guilty because no proper action has been undertaken.

The mental health burden is heavy and may not be worth what we are doing to our children and seniors. Despite COVID-19 restrictions, many of us found ways to celebrate Hannukah, Christmas, the Western, and the Lunar (Chinese) New Year, spreading holiday cheer inside the family using online platforms. Still, this celebration was missing in many families on social support, fragmentary internet connection, and domestic episodes of abuse. Several youths are on suicide watch, and the burden of post-traumatic stress disorder is still underestimated. The current coronavirus pandemic is still raging on with variants, and vaccination supplies may not go to cover any single corner of the entire planet. New variants seem to harbor more contagiousness and may weaken the efficacy of some vaccines. The risk of continuing the infection for a couple of more years is not unjustified without successful herd immunity. In different conversations, people talk about their emotional distress, and there is a growing sense of despair mixed with several notes of surrealism. There are evident mental health issues, and researchers found increased depression and anxiety stemming from the pandemic. However, some experts argue that it may not be the actual root of the problem [272]. Scapegoating the coronavirus for the current mental health issues may be too simplistic. Months of restrictions, isolation, virtual education, and uncertainty are taking a heavy toll on the emotional well-being of increasing numbers of people. It has become an everyday routine to medicalize human suffering. We do it by assigning a mental health diagnosis to it, but the source of people's anguish is not addressed. The virus creates mental attitudes and habits in several individuals unable to deny some of the pandemic conditions that may be challenging to accept. Several youths are unable to cope and adapt, originating connotations from their own experiences. We need to name our experiences. It matters how we make sense of our distress. Our human nature develops a process of avoidance and denial, often involuntarily, to protect us from the more worrying parts of our lives. We believe in the certainty of tomorrow and deny the inevitability of death by promoting illusions of confidence and the immortal presence with avatars in social platforms. Our minds can accept and usually tolerate short periods of ambiguity, but prolonged periods trigger denial and mental health issues. The current pandemic has been jabbing at the defense mechanisms many individuals and families rely on just to create a sense of stability. This pandemic has left several individuals and families feeling emotionally exposed and unprotected. The terrifying practice of medicalizing human suffering has become routine with an increase in anxiolytic drug use.

Emotional well-being relies on a sense of equilibrium. The "yin and yang" equilibrium is vital in understanding the importance of well-being. The individual's ability to preserve and, if poked, restore equilibrium relies on how we can make sense of our experiences. Disequilibrium is the natural consequence when we experience the burden of accumulated adversities. The vulnerability to disequilibrium is associated with suffering. To remedy anguish and misery, it is common to search for scapegoats. Virtual meeting fatigue is a symptom of our electronic overconnection. Despite being useful, it may be inappropriate for interpersonal relationships. It is even more challenging for several individuals to remain connected to the sense of mutual human understanding that anchors the customary. The Power Threat Meaning Framework is a tool to clarify and highlight the interrelated connection between social and experiential factors affecting the subjective nature of emotional suffering [175]. In the absence of weekly or monthly sacramentary reconciliation due to the restriction to church services, this tool may help in re-identifying the equilibrium. It is paramount to normalize responses to adversity rather than medicalize them, but obviously, it is also a matter of cost. Human interconnection setup has a high monetary value than prescribing anxiolytic drugs. The Power Threat Meaning Framework suggests five practical elements for coping with complicated feelings during the pandemic. It is crucial that we focus on the approach to be present. Our experience needs to be free of pre-judgment. Also, secondly, basic elements remain essential and include healthy nutrition, good sleep, daily indoor or outdoor physical activity, and safe socialization striving for a work-life balance. A 3rd element is a search for a balance between acknowledging the experiences in which the hope for better humanity starts in the single individuum. They are far more fundamental and fertile than despair and worrying facts. Also, structuring daily life is crucial because it is a friendly approach to adversity. Finally, asking for help takes courage, and, in an individualistic society, it may be challenging. A 6th point may concern rebranding community services with primary divine consideration of human fragility. There are several challenges to humanity, and the extinction can start from inside us and will not be a catastrophic climatic event. There is a significant challenge more devastating than COVID-19 to our society and is not terrorism or climate change, but there is an indiscriminate attack on the nucleus of our community. Climate change is an emergency, but the attack on the family is a much more emergency because if we destroy the family, we will exhaust the planet.

Self-indulgence is an actual danger for our countries. The opioid crisis is a dread to our civilization. Education and perseverance in the fight against self-indulgence will be key. Currently, the COVID-19 pandemic has fueled the rate of lives we lost to the opioid crisis. The dramatic pace of over 81,000 drug overdose deaths in the United States in the 12 months ending in May 2020, which was the highest number of overdose deaths ever recorded in 12 months, according to recent provisional data from the Centers for Disease Control and Prevention (CDC) [273] is abysmal and appalling. According to CDC, there has been an obvious acceleration of such deaths during the pandemic and lockdowns. If we add the suicides, it is excruciating. The struggle of the most vulnerable layers of our society has not been understood. Synthetic opioids (primarily illicitly manufactured fentanyl, either coming nationally or from foreign countries) appear to be the main driver of the surges in overdose deaths. Fentanyl is a powerful synthetic opioid with a chemical structure and pharmaceutical action like morphine but is 50 to 100 times more potent [274, 275]. Fentanyl has an enormous burden on our society. Fentanyl is habitually used to take care of patients experiencing severe pain, particularly after surgery [276]. It is also occasionally used to treat patients with chronic pain who became physically tolerant to other opioids. However, the culprit seems to be the illicit fentanyl and heroin use and not the opioid analgesic prescription. The sharp overdose recorded in 2014 was driven by illegal fentanyl and heroin. According to Rose [277], only 3.6% of individuals initiate heroin use within five years of initial prescription opioid misuse. Even though the United States consumes 80% of the world's opioid supply, opioid access is nonexistent in four out of five individuals and restricted to about one to twenty individuals of the global population. However, opioid analgesic prescribing needs to be revised to balance the potential benefit for patients in need of these drugs. Substantially, there has been an escalating 38.4% from the 12 months leading up to June 2019 contrasting sharply the 12 months up to May 2020. Overdose deaths involving cocaine also increased by 26.5%. These deaths have been linked to co-use or contamination of cocaine with illicitly manufactured fentanyl or other drugs, such as heroin. Overdose deaths involving psychostimulants, such as methamphetamine, increased sharply and shockingly by 34.8%. The CDC recommendations include the expansion of distribution and use of naloxone, overdose prevention education, and early intervention of individuals at highest risk for overdose are not satisfactory. These recommendations do not tackle the opioid crisis at the root. The disaggregation of the youth, the weakening of the conservative values, the tolerance to racist actions, the poor education, and the erosion of public trust are also important aspects to ponder. Although opioids are illegal in some foreign countries, some chemists are skilled at developing new analogs. Their companies can sell these legally on the internet without penalties, staying a step forward of the governments, and local authorities do not favor an industrial decline or control in this sector because it is substantially an economical source for thousands of unethical chemical companies [278]. However, it is easy to culprit any country or company because there is a demand for fentanyl and illicit drugs in the industrialized world. Further, many less scrupulous individuals cooperate to the vitality and support of this supply chain. Thus, we need to tackle educating our youth and future generations about the danger of self-indulgence. We will need to increase the budget, techniques, and strategies of the Drug Enforcement Administration (DEA) and similar agencies worldwide to combat drug trafficking and distribution within the US more effectively and efficiently.

Odysseus, also known as Ulysses, covered his ears to avoid being enchanting by the sirens' attracting and mortal song. The Sirens were creatures from Greek mythology which enticed sailors to their destruction with their irresistibly beautiful singing. Their most famous appearance in literature is Homer's Odyssey, where the hero Odysseus, on his long voyage home following the Trojan War, successfully escapes their enchanting call. Using a block of beeswax, a gift of Circe, Odysseus was able to adapt some fragments of it in the ears of his co-sailors, who left them prepared to the temptation of the song of the Sirens. Still, he had to stoically survive this time by letting his companions tie him firmly to the ship's mast. The beautiful but noxious song dulcifies Odysseus's heart, letting his sailors order to let him free. Although the Sirens look as beautiful as Helen of Troy to Odysseus, who is bewitched by the fraudulent and mellifluous song, they appear in their entirety as hungry monsters with crooked claws to his sailors. Odysseus was saved by his humility in accepting the advice of the goddess Circe. Odysseus will go through many more temptations and trials before he can finally reach his home and family. Engaging in addictive behavior is easy for humans for both biological and evolutionary reasons. The key to regaining our freedom is resolution, determination, and self-control. In planning like Odysseus, the plan to increase our self-control goes into the decision of strategy. It starts identifying the danger or the perilous moments when the lure is stranger and the motivation is lower. It continues in identifying our crew or our friends meticulously. It is essential to realize that it is audacious to stop indulging when our friends or staff indulge in such behavior. Knowing our ship or environment is also the next step in understanding where our self-control will be lessened. Similar to Odysseus, we need to be willing to accept and execute the plan until the end. We may suffer like Odysseus, but his sacrifice was not in vain because the Sirens were fated to die if a mortal could escape them after hearing them singing. Self-indulgence kills our humility and our freedom. It is not the way of the perfect world of which the imitation speaks, but the road that leads to perfection. Sanctity does not consist of extraordinary things but in doing ordinary things systematically and exceptionally well.

Marijuana is illegal in numerous countries and the United States of America under federal law. It is classified as a Schedule I drug in the Controlled Substances Act (CSA), alongside heroin. In general, cannabis describes cannabis products. Marijuana explicitly refers to cannabis products that are produced from the dried flowers, leaves, stems, and, of course, seeds of the cannabis plant. The current classification says that the substances have no entirely accepted medicinal value. Some benefit has been given to cannabis for some diseases, e.g., multiple sclerosis-related spasticity, nausea and vomiting caused by chemotherapy, appetite loss associated with certain types of cancers, and neuropathic pain. However, the science remains inconclusive on the health effects of prolonged use of cannabis. It does not rule out that in single cases, this product may be beneficial. In reality, cannabis bears mostly a heavy burden to our society ahead. Its legalization can put down the morale of the nations, and the sufferance of Chinese people during the opium wars is memorable and emblematic. The potential release of the symptoms of some diseases has been highly provocative and debatable. It seems to percept a surrogate of the fight against prohibition like the historical prohibition against alcohol of the last century. However, cannabis is far from being like alcohol. Marijuana may undermine the health of second-hand smokers, like tobacco users in both family households and fraternities. The legalization of recreational use will decrease the ability to discerning medical users effectively. The most meticulous screening and vulnerable police check cannot completely rule out the infiltration of criminal enterprises. These companies can set up ways to control legal shops and use the legally received financial support to finance illegal activities. Also, the "safe" impression derived from a legal use after 18 or 21 years will give children and adolescents the impression that its use is comparable safe to tobacco in youth. It has been easily demonstrated the variety of setbacks in the young teens' experience from using marijuana. The measurement and assessment of impaired driving under cannabis influence or post-smoking are still imprecise and easy to manipulate much better than alcohol because of the different catabolic substances. It is unpredictable the spiral that may be evoked when legalization will lead to a surge in use, compounding already high rates of substance use worldwide. There is more in considering the cons of using cannabis because frequent marijuana use can seriously affect short-term memory, impair cognitive ability, lung tissue elasticity, induce cancer, and carry a risk of abuse and addiction. The damage to the hippocampus is quite concerning. A study published by Northwestern University in the journal "*Hippocampus*" showed, through MRIs, an oddly shaped hippocampus in

16 and 17-years-old adolescents who had used marijuana for three years [279]. The hippocampus is the brain region most responsible for short- and long-term memory. This pathological finding is not surprising considering the abnormal cognitive abilities of cannabis users. The side effects are not trivial and may include more substantial anxiety, hallucinations, palpitations, and vasodilatation. It may trigger schizophrenia and other psychiatric disorders, e.g., bipolar disorders, in vulnerable individuals. Myclobutanil ("Eagle 20") is a fungicide used by several pot cultivators and grape growers and may turn into hydrogen cyanide when heated. Although grapes get washed and crashed, cannabis gets harvested, dried, and sold, wehere cannabis is primarily heated, and inhaled, increasing the unhealthy burden on consumers. In Canada and some US states, the use of cannabis for medicinal purposes and partially for recreational use has been legalized. However, it will need more moves by policymakers and the US government for it to be accepted and sold nationwide. The benefits of having it for a few medical symptoms and diseases must be balanced and weighted with the negative effect on the cognitive ability of youth and future adult generations. Some data would suggest that the introduction of legalized recreational cannabis may lead to some decline in opioid-related deaths, but public health and politicians are misleading our society. Is it not the reason for medicine to look for the cause of disease and not promoting new symptomatic therapies? We should search why opioid use is not safe and how the abuse can be better prevented rather proposing another remedy that will debilitate the future generations to come. It is immoral to think about profits using dubious substances. In Colorado, for example, nearly $200 million in tax revenue was collected in 2016 on just over $1.3 billion in legal sales. Other states are contemplating the recreational-pot industry as a measure to re-start the economy after the current pandemic. There is a genuine and grounded concern that younger adults could see their brains adversely affected using marijuana. The long-term impact on the brain, lungs, and other organs is not known enough. Since teenagers are the most vulnerable population, we, as physicians, need to act. Teenagers may not consider lowering intelligence quotient or cognitive ability a dramatic effect because the sensation of

wellness it procures is relaxing and fun, so they do not care about the product's danger.

Opium Wars left a deep scar on the collective conscience of the Chinese culture, which bans any recreation drugs altogether. Although it may be considered excessive, it is correct and has connections and roots with the damages suffered by Chinese people fighting Western imperialism. The Chinese aversion against opium and recreating drugs have similar aspects with the Christian Heritage. It has been often documented the sacrality of the body in the correspondence of the Christian Fathers and Proto-Christians. The indulgence of the human spirit with such drugs may have a severe deviation of the personality, and ignoring these aspects will inevitably leave our body and soul to corruption. Marihuana is highly prone to addiction and more than we thought in the '80s and '90s. New evidence suggests that marijuana legalization leads to more cannabis use and perhaps frank addiction. Long-term or heavy use of cannabis products is linked to psychological and physical health concerns, lower educational attainment, inescapabledecline in social class, unemployment, and motor vehicle crashes. These effects are not trivial, considering the devastating impact of the ongoing pandemic. Marijuana remains a drug that does not contribute to the level of humanity or culture in a nation. It remains and should remain an illicit drug worldwide, not because big pharma companies support other drugs but because of users' psychology. Potentially, second-hand users are highly affected. Although the percentual increase is not dramatic, the current trend with deprivation of school teaching would profoundly affect the youth aspiration and career. The prominent role the United States and Canada will play in the future is at stake. In legalization states, older adults classified past-month use increased and there was also a relative increase in cannabis use disorder among adolescents. No matter how small data are, the failure to protect youth will be considered irresponsible in the centuries to come. Although climate change is an emergency, the failure to tackle the illicit use of opioids, cannabis, or other illegal drugs will frail and destroy our roots. As states are proceeding to legalize marijuana, we need to measure public health effects closely, but the results could be devastating. Since every child matters, physicians are paramount to banning all drugs altogether and regulating opioid prescription. However, it is not enough. We need to target education and re-educate our generations about the importance of alternatives to drugs for recreation or pain control. If a person is anxious, anxiolytic drugs are not the answer. We need to identify the roots that provoke anxiety, and drug-free therapies have been considered successful. The future of our youth remains exclusively in our hands, and promoting liberal, disgraceful, and fraudolent concepts will inevitably destroy our communities and our society. Of course, we can concentrate on our community and consider other communities' troubles a remote event, but this approach will lead to a more crackled society. Numerous legal actions need to be considered now to target destructive patterns of our nations [280-289].

Anti-family legislations and political feelings against the traditional family have been perpetuated for the last ten lustra ripping apart the family as emphasized in the core of the American and Canadian Great Fathers. Although debated, we continue to live in an era of profound aversion towards the family, both at the ideological level and at the level of real life, as highlighted recently [290]. It is a continuous and subdulous aggression that affects the cultural level first and the Free Speech Rights. There is a political and cultural process that has gradually eroded the centrality of the family worldwide to the point of explicit adversity. There is an environment of erroneous principles and false attitudes of the current society that exalts more individualism and community and less concerning the family. There is an atmosphere of disbelief, accompanied by a denial of religion, with its precepts and sanctions, to generate a cruel apostasy from the supernatural of entire nations. Prof. Toniolo suggests that "The protection, the restoration, the elevation of the family, must today be assumed not as a task of a few and more fervent representatives of private and social interests, but as a work of common salvation and civilization " [291]. The Mexican civil war of the 1920s is an example to consider. The *Cristiada* was a popular counter-revolution, genuinely spontaneous and autonomous. The *Cristiada* was victorious, and the *Cristeros*, the men, armed with pistols and crosses, who fought the socialist government of Plutarch Calles from 1925 to 1929, did not want power. They want to preserve the Catholic faith. Mexican Catholics of the time were often described as backward people having obscurantist tendencies. Still, its leaders were laypeople, priests, and workers, fathers, mothers, daughters, and sons who defended their right to receive the sacraments, made impossible by the totalitarian laws of Calles. The assault on the family did not begin in the contestations of the '60s and '70s, but it is more than two centuries old, starting with modernism views, which slowly invaded our societies. Currently, we are facing a legislative and juridical direction in which the fundamental cell of society is about to be transformed into a mere sum of individuals. There is a continuous attack toward the traditional family. Giuseppe Toniolo was a professor who spent his life fighting for the family's sacrality [291]. The importance of understanding the Lord's presence in our world is critical. In our societies' current anti-family legislation and political actions, there is continuous promulgation of individualistic laws. Thus, the individual becomes fatally de-centered and disconnected, progressively experiencing solitude, anxiety, and depression.

Humility and its practice may be the roots. The Fathers of the Canadian Confederation and the Fathers of the American Constitution may have left some footsteps that we may need to follow again and emulate. Our Fathers were not perfect but they had the traditional family in mind. We need to learn to practice humility, which is necessary for prayerful souls and glorifying the dignity of the human being as Divine creation. Humility needs to be acquired with constant prayer, charity, and mortification. It is important to learn to practice humility on every occasion. It may help in the war against recreational drugs and rejuvenate the human spirit fighting the mental health issues we face during this pandemic and the post-traumatic disorder we may face in the next few years. Humility was present in the Fathers who supported the Canadian Confederation and the American Constitution. Humility is the key to identifying ways to improve the social needs in our society and divine contemplation. Humility is also key for fighting self-indulgence, which is a poison for the body and the soul. We are not delighted in mortifying ourselves, and practicing humility needs a lot of work. The body is imperfect, and the more we give, the more it requires [292]. In each conversion, it is important to find a spiritual guide. The spiritual path can be identified with quietness and tranquility. In this conversion (or reconversion), listening to the silence and Divinity is crucial, but such predisposition requires a progressive detachment from the world. Such a track does not need to be physical because the individual still needs to use several media to communicate but gradually considers the true importance of such social communication in life. In this progressive distancing, which is not different from weighing such social media opportunities, there is the opportunity to increase the introspection of the own soul. It is important to take care of and take the most outstanding care of our souls. Our world is frequently keen to disavow the soul. *Inimici hominis domestici eius* (ἐχθροὶ τοῦ ἀνθρώπου οἱ οἱκιακοὶ αὑτοῦ) (Matthew 10:36) [184], which means a man's servants are his enemies or better flatmates rather than servants or relatives. We need to remember the vanity of all things and of how quickly they pass away. There is a vulnerability in keeping ephemeral things attached to our hearts. Pride and super-righteousness are destructive. Mortification is hard to conquer. It may mean collecting the toilet paper on the ground of a public washroom before the janitor comes to clean it. Pride destroys individuals, families, and nations. In His preaching in the Sermon of the Mount, it is admonished that "Blessed are the poor in spirit, for theirs is the kingdom of heaven" (Matthew 5:3) [184]. Solomon's words lay caution against choosing to sin deliberately. Sin is very addictive, and criminology schools, as well as scientific reports, have identified this relationship incredibly early [293]. The firmness of character needs to be praised. Humility and mortification fortify the character of men and women. They are a "*conditio sine qua non*" to taste the sweetness in all bitterness and to encourage to escape the promiscuous and mischievous "Land of Egypt." The opportunity to act anytime in the Divine presence is a good way of keeping ourselves away from trouble [292]. It is important not to judge when we are strong, when the Divine Strength gave us tremendous fortitude, but assess ourselves in our weakest moments of our life. Constance and vigilance are a must to continue humility as indicated in the sentence "*vigilate itaque omni tempore orantes*" suggesting to be alert at any time avoiding that pride reaches our soul (Luke XX1, 36) [294].

Prayer is an essential aspect of our life, and the Fathers of the American nation knew how important it is. The Establishing Fathers of the United

States of America were American and devoted leaders not without sin but united to build the most glorious nation the world ever had. They connected the Thirteen Colonies leading without selfishness the war for independence from England. Fear was present, but also courage and humility. They built a frame of government for the United States of America upon republican principles. In 1973, historian Richard B. Morris identified the following seven figures as key Great Fathers: John Adams, Benjamin Franklin, Alexander Hamilton, John Jay, Thomas Jefferson, James Madison, and George Washington [295]. His analysis based on the critical and substantive roles the Fathers played in forming the country's new government has been to reinstate the importance of the United States of America for the concept of democracy in the Western world. The United States of America and Canada are not perfect and our past has missteps that need to be rectified. But the "cancel culture" is not the answer. In the 18th century until 1962, it was common practice for public schools in the United States to have an open prayer or Bible reading. In a 1962 decision, the US Supreme Court prohibited school-sponsored prayer in public schools. The former US president was an active supporter of the religious freedom but also identified that it is deleterious when the State interposes between the individual and the Divine. The Supreme Court has never outlawed "prayer in schools" but the sentence was often misinterpreted. In fact, pupils or students can pray alone or in groups, as long as such activities are not obstructive and do not infringe upon the right of other pupils or students. Interstingly, 1962 is also the year of the Second Vatican Council, which not only approved the change of the language of the liturgy from Latin into vernacular that may be perfectly understandable, but changed deeply the liturgy with the priest not any more prone to the Tabernacle but facing the audience in an act, which may be considered irreverent according to the Old Testament. Teresa d'Avila mentions how important it is to pray [292]. Praying without interruption and meditation day and night. After prayer, Teresa d'Avila mentions fasting, penances, and silence. All are part of the same dimension to reach spiritual virtues and lead communities. True prayer is crucial and helps us preserve the unity of the individuum, the family, and the nation. Three things help in the prayer, and all of them are of the same dimension.

They include 1) love for one another, 2) detachment from all created things and unnecessary tools of our life, and 3) perseverance in humility. Here it is also briefly essential to mention David and Goliah. As indicated in the biblical Book of Samuel, the young David defeated the Philistine giant in single combat. David was fearless and had only a sling and a pouch full of stones against Goliath's sword and shield. Although Goliath was attacking and killing, David found a weak spot in his opponent's armor. David slung one of his stones in the vulnerable site and, knocking him out. David won the war for the Israelites. Although the story is referenced as a moral lesson of how underdogs can overcome the odds and be subsequently successful, it allows analyzing four features of his strategy that may be useful in science, politics, business, sports, and life. The four features of David's strategy include 1) speed and agility, 2) accuracy, 3) assessment of odds and 4) sagacity in the choice of action. Goliath was big and robust, while David was quick and agile. Speed and agility are crucial in any action, mainly when the odds are against us. Speed and agility can become highly advantageous. The advantage of this agility by learning and failing fast, reacting swiftly, and changing can become crucial for the final win. Accuracy matters because David precisely identified a vulnerable spot where he could effectively fight against Goliath. The appropriate disruption of common sense and odds relies on how we can overcome the odds and subsequently succeed. The sagacity of the line of action indicates our continuous training with modern and easy tools to use and keep with us. The choice of a great equalizer is critical for a victory. Health disparities have plagued both the United States and Canada and deeply impacted racial and ethnic minorities. Despite COVID-19 places everyone at risk, we need to realize that it is not "the great equalizer" because it has targeted and continues to target the socially disadvantaged layers of our societies [296]. Thus, it is our responsibility as physicians to pinpoint and alter these outcomes for our patients. Humility is rarely taught today. Numerous mystics and visionaries contributed enormously to the diffusion of Christianity. St. Teresa of Avila, St. Hildegard of Bingen, and St. Catherine of Genoa are a few of them that left a footstep in the book of humility. Teresa of Avila was a Discalced Carmelite nun who founded a reformed monastery and wrote the *Camino de*

Perfección or the Way of Perfection in the 16th century. Discalced Carmelites have roots in the eremitic traditions of the Catholic Church. Teresa was a key personality of the Counter-Reformation. She taught her nuns how to progress through prayer and Christian meditation. She described how to attain spiritual perfection through prayer in four stages: meditation, quiet, repose of soul, and finally, perfect union with the Lord. Her book was painting the fight of any form of self-indulgence graphically, leaving the human spirit able to reach the Divine Presence [292]. A few centuries earlier, an essential step in favor of humility was spent by Hildegard of Bingen [297]. She lived from 1098 to 1179, suggesting a way to experience the same vision she had, demanding a journey beyond our self-pre-occupation and into a genuine friendship with the Divine Presence, a company protected by the strength of the Divine Justice. Corporal and spiritual indulgences may leave the human soul able to be raped by our temptations, and addiction is an often-identified peril in our humanity. A similar approach to gaining humility is suggested by Catherine Benincasa, who. in 1353, at the of 6 years, experienced the first of the mystical visions that would power her extraordinary life. St. Catherine's piety was immense. In imitating the public flagellants who had been roaming Europe since the outbreak of bubonic plague, Catherine reinvigorated her spirit by fighting self-indulgence. In all three female stories, there is austerity without any mitigation. There is religious observance and recollection, unceasing prayer, and as much labor as human nature can bear. It is essential to reflect on the practice of prayer and meditation of the three saints. Their mortification should inspire our generation and future generations about the right approach to self-will. All things that bring us far from the Divinity and Creator are vanity and ephemeral. It seems that we echo Luke (22:15 Ἐπιθυμίᾳ ἐπεθύμησα τοῦτο τὸ πάσχα φαγεῖν μεθ' ὑμῶν πρὸ τοῦ με παθεῖν, which means with hunger, I hunger for this, the Passover. In all three saints, the fear of the Lord is sublime. Our actions need to be considered cautiously and seriously, trying to keep things and persons away that bring us far from the Lord. It is crucial to avoid "theo-fugal" cultures. We can still be anthropocentric but keeping "theo-centricity" is an essential premise for love and eternity. Theocentric love is anthropocentric when florid and fertile, while the "theo-fugal" love is "anthropo-fugal" when it is arid, wordy, and leaving us without fruits. In this sense, all three mystical women expressed a pure theocentric love, which is part of the itinerary to the full contemplation and continuous adoration of the Divinity into the Blessed Sacrament. However, an essential and "treacherous" temptation is the feeling of confidence. Thus, mortification and humility are the critical milestones for an ordinary life with extraordinary attachment to the Divinity. A minimalist approach with frugality was the mainstay. The firm determination to forgive our debtors is a necessary premise to start the full contemplation of the Lord. Even it is not sufficient. It is essential and compulsory to place our souls far from credits to avoid the illusions and delights that we are holy and worthy of tremendous honor. Humility is our safeguard and treating everybody with respect as in Divine presence. True humility never disquiets nor bothers the soul, but irenic, peaceful, and sweet. We need to respect even the iota of the Torah, and the importance of being in communion with the Lord is key because our body is a temple of God. Thus, be irreverent with our body would incite irreverence to the Creator.

Heritage is in each of us, and we need to re-awake our spirit to avoid losing our freedom forever. It is up to us which root we will take, but our responsibility is for the Fathers to keep the American Dream vivid. Yes, we can, we can cover our ears like Odysseus, close our eyes and go away of the danger of the evil, but we need to choose our friends, to check the ship and the frame that we use to sail or drive, and be stack to the program, which can be arduous and excruciating. St. Teresa d' Avila reminds us to care nothing for any earthly pain when there is a question of rendering some more extraordinary service to the Creator, who suffered for us. Those who are over-anxious about what will be given them will, someday or other, out of custom, ask for what they do not want and perhaps from people more ready than themselves. Poverty includes all good things in this world and all advantages of modern life. Poverty is a vast domain and requires a meek and humble heart to appreciate it. Longings, cravings, lust, and desires can be mortal if not correctly addressed. An aspiration for honor and loyalty always carries with it some regard for poverty. There is a lot of literature to limit Big Tech's intrusion into the lives of our generations, and there is a need now for American families to discredit Big Tech for violating the interests of minors. Teresa d' Avila inspired mates, students, parents, neighbors, brothers and sisters to be closer to the Lord. She commented how the Church needed to become a place of adoration and prayer again and not a place to incite and bind political and business favors. In the 16th century, when St. Teresa d' Avila wrote her book, tremendous heresies brought to the destruction of Catholic churches, profanation of the Sacraments, the mayhem of sacred images, havoc, and sacking of convents, and perpetual murder of priests and nuns. The iconoclastic behavior and destruction of traditional values happened again in our century and started progressively following the failure of capitalism without humanism. She fought like St. Ambrose when she condemned many mischievous aspects surrounding the Church at the end of the 4th century. Both Teresa d'Avila and Ambrose are only two of the numerous examples of people requiring renewal of the Church and their societies. The current pandemic and the excruciating rates of drug-related deaths and suicides demand a radical renewal of our societies.

Chapter 8

VACCINES AND WARP

ABSTRACT

This chapter presents some factual vaccine information and some aspects of the WARP speed operation, which has been conducted to rapid develop of vaccines against SARS-CoV-2.

Keywords: vaccines, WARP, biotechnology

Vaccines are powerful against dangerous infections, from Jenner's cowpox to messenger RNA (mRNA) COVID-19 vaccines. Numerous children and adults have been saved over the years since vaccine inception. However, low socio-economic countries may be in trouble if we do not consider vaccine equality [298]. Currently, the vaccines in use are based on the type of active component. They are discerned in live attenuated virus vaccines, inactivated or virus-killed vaccines, subunit vaccines, and recombinant DNA/RNA vaccines. The live attenuated vaccines are produced from microorganisms declared non-pathogenic (e.g., measles, mumps, rubella viruses). The inactivated (or virus-killed) vaccines are produced from microorganisms inactivated. It means the microorganisms are killed by exposure to heat or chemical substances (e.g., hepatitis A virus and poliomyelitis). The subunit vaccines are produced through refined purification techniques of the antigenic components of the pathogen and its toxins (e.g., pertussis or whooping cough, meningitis, tetanus, and diphtheria). In contrast, the recombinant DNA/mRNA genetic vaccines are linked to the most recent biotechnological procedures. The recombinant DNA/mRNA genetic vaccines are produced from portions of the microorganism's genome. This part of the viral genome codes for a certain antigen is crucial for the pathogenesis of the infection. A biotechnology-based process uses viral transport vectors. These vectors carry the instructions to make neutralizing antibodies. The immune cells will set the specific antibody response against this antigen (e.g., vaccines for hepatitis B virus and meningococcus B). Vaccines can also be distinguished from the active components that they contain. Thus, we can have monovalent vaccines containing only one antigen preventing only one disease. Multivalent vaccines include several antigens for the prevention of several diseases at the same time. Vaccines can also be differentiated depending on the route of administration (e.g., subcutaneous, intramuscular, oral, and inhalation – nasal spray). The use of biotechnology has been largely used against the SARS-CoV-2. The genetic vaccines against the current pandemic use mRNA. The information enters the individual's cells to produce the spike protein, which the coronavirus uses to bind human cells and penetrate them. The vaccines based on mRNA different from conventional vaccines do not result from a growth in eggs or cells, which may also have important ethical and religious implications. The biotechnology based on these unconventional vaccines allows a fast development showing an immunological benefit. These mRNA vaccines seem to add to the stimulation of antibodies and helper T lymphocytes that bear the CD4 antigen (CD, cluster of differentiation) and the activation of cytotoxic T lymphocytes, which bear the CD8 antigen. This bold activation occurs using the major histocompatibility complex (MHC), which is a large genetic locus containing a set of polymorphic genes able to code for cell surface proteins. These proteins are essential for the adaptive immune system. The mRNA vaccines, issued by Pfizer-BioNTech (BNT162b2) and Moderna (mRNA-1273), do not employ preformed viruses to deliver the antigen in the individual's body. This technology is different from the traditional technology as seen in the AstraZeneca vaccine, which uses a modified adenovirus to carry parts of SARS-CoV-2 capable of stimulating the immune response. In traditional technology, a hybrid adenovirus-coronavirus is assembled, stimulating the production of antibodies to both viruses. The advantage of mRNA vaccines is that the individual's immune system produces antibodies more efficiently and effectively. On the other side, despite some vaccine-induced thrombophilia, the UK massive deployment of the AstraZeneca vaccine has gained success worldwide with minimal side effects. It may be needed to digress at this stage, informing that some minimal or mild symptoms may occur with all vaccines. This is due to the local and systemic reaction of the immune system to a foreign body being inoculated into the body. The production of specific neutralizing antibodies capable of protecting the host and understanding circulating immune memory for SARS-CoV-2 in case of re-exposure is key. In patients who contracted the COVID-19, the Spike-IgG (immunoglobulin G) antibody titer was found to be stable for over six months. Also, B lymphocytes bearing a specific memory and able to produce immunoglobulins were more copious at six months than at one month after infection. T cells bearing the cluster of differentiation 4 and 8 or CD4 + and T CD8 + lymphocytes specific for SARS-CoV2 showed a half-life of 3-5 months [299]. Widge et al. (2021) showed that the developed mRNA-1273 vaccine from Moderna Biotech induced elevated levels of neutralizing specific antibodies, which decreased quite slightly over time. The authors suggest that the mRNA-1273 vaccine can provide lasting and unfluctuating humoral immunity in a way better than that conferred by natural infection [300]. The risks raised by the skepticism of biotechnology that the host DNA may be mutated are groundless. Unfortunately, fake news and vaccine hesitancy /refusal group papers have circulated on social media and major newspapers and television broadcasts, raising concerns and doubts about the full process [301]. Crucial is that the mRNA cannot cause infection, unlike the virus, since it does not penetrate the cell nucleus. Also, it cannot integrate into the nuclear DNA of host cells. The mRNA has an extremely low half-time and needs to be kept at low temperatures for transportation before being inoculated. The mRNA following translation to code proteins must be degraded with its lipid carrier. The new technology may be crucial for developing potential vaccines against several other infectious agents and, probably, against cancer. It has been auspicated that a new personalized vaccine may generate precise immune responses when administered with a drug adjuvant (e.g., a checkpoint inhibitor) to effectively reduce the tumor size [302, 303].

Public-private partnerships have been key to tackle several health issues in the past. Public-private partnerships are not uncommon in business and represent an agreement to generate income or human development using a formal cooperation between public institutions and private companies. Both public and private sectors made tremendous investments in global health over the past several decades. These partnerships (e.g., the Bill and Melinda Gates Foundation) have been crucial for setting up and starting to tackle diseases in health programs, such as child and maternal health, malaria, and HIV [304]. Operation Warp Speed (OWS) is such a formidable public-private partnership. It has been initiated by the US government to facilitate and accelerate the development, manufacturing, and distribution of COVID-19 diagnostics, therapeutics, and vaccines. Although the first news report of OWS took place on April 29th, 2020 [299, 302, 303], the program was officially declared on May 15th, 2020. One of the most important tasks carried out by OWS was the production of multiple vaccines through different types of vaccine technologies. OWS gave paths to allow a faster distribution of vaccines against SARS-CoV-2 if clinical trials would confirm one or more vaccines would be safe and effective. The former US president Donald Trump facilitated the creation of OWS, which was initially funded with about $10 billion from the CARES Act (Coronavirus Aid, Relief, and Economic Security). The Congress passed this Act on March 27, 2020. The CARES Act is an interagency program that includes several Department of Health and Human Services components. It includes the National Institutes of Health, the Centers for Disease Control and Prevention, the Food and Drug Administration, the Biomedical Advanced Research and Development Authority (BARDA), the Department of Defense, and private firms. Other federal agencies, including the Department of Veterans Affairs, the Department of Energy, and the Department of Agriculture, , also contributed to the program supported by the CARES Act. Although the new administration is reluctant to use it, the utilization of Warp Speed's name to the partnership was inspired by the faster-than-light travel used in the Star Trek fictional universe. It supported and motivated both public and private sector arousing a sense of rapid progress for the current pandemic. OWS included eight firms, including Johnson & Johnson (Janssen Pharmaceutical), which used the non-replicating viral vector (Ad26.COV2-S), the AstraZeneca–University of Oxford/Vaccitech, which used a modified chimpanzee adenovirus viral vector (AZD1222), Moderna the mRNA technology (mRNA-1273), Novavax a SARS-CoV-2 recombinant spike protein nanoparticle with adjuvant (NVX-CoV2373), Merck and IAVI targeting antiviral drug research and immune response therapy, Sanofi and GlaxoSmithKline using the protein on insect cell lines and an adjuvant. Indirectly funded companies included Inovio, Regeneron, and Vaxart, , while a company that has not received OWS funding was Pfizer-BioNTech to the best of my knowledge. Yet, this firm received some funding from the government of Germany to accelerate the development and production capacity of the vaccine. An outcry took place in France for the inefficiency to rollout vaccines, particularly for the huge role the Institute Pasteur played in the microbiology, public health, and development of vaccines in the past. Although Canada's rollout can be understood for failed policies and defective regulation, France's rollout remains highly embarrassing, as highlighted recently in *Le Figaro*, and many suggest the rate of vaccine hesitancy due to the use of a foreign vaccine [305]. Considering the enormous contribution to vaccines and immunology in general France has deployed in the last centuries, it should be considered a failure for President Macron's government. However, it would be inappropriate to identify the current French President as the culprit of the situation. This attitude bears the responsibility to varying degrees with French failed scientific and political programs of the last two-three decades.

Chapter 9

VACCINES FAILURE, HESITANCY, AND REFUSAL

ABSTRACT

This chapter deals with the drama of the run for a COVID-19 vaccine. Vaccine hesitancy and refusal generated by the misunderstanding of immunology and politics have become substantial obstacles to reach a satisfactory herd immunity. Currently, misinformation about vaccines can ultimately jeopardize the success of the fight against COVID-19. Reluctance and even refusal are granted in several constitutions as human rights but may constitute a danger for the solution of the current pandemic. The safety and efficacy of vaccines are presented.

Keywords: vaccines, failure, hesitancy, refusal

Vaccine failure may be treacherous for humanity, and all parties need to work together to maximize the population. Vaccines are efficacious, and compelling and early data identify an impressive protection rate for some countries [306]. In Israel, which, to the best of our knowledge, has the highest rate of COVID-19 vaccination worldwide, public health indicators support and praise the impact of the vaccination program. The mRNA-based vaccine seems to prevent 94% of symptomatic infections, confirming that this vaccine performs just as well in a larger community as it did in the clinical trials. It was crucial to vaccinate the most susceptible groups. This new technology-based vaccine prevented almost all cases of serious illness. These are formidable news considering the "speed" at which this product was manufactured. The roughly 94% rate seems to be the same in all age groups, including the septuagenarians and over. These age groups may have been under-represented in the original clinical trials used to approve the vaccine. The message seems to be clear that there is a solid need to get "very high" coverage of the risk groups. These individuals are most probably the subjects that may become extremely ill from the coronavirus. The initial criticisms against Israel for the Palestinian communities seem unjustified because Israel had already started to transfer some doses to Palestinians in the West Bank and Gaza. Lockdown measures were relieved, and education re-started. Nevertheless, vaccines may fail to reach herd immunity worldwide, and six factors can contribute to this failure. Some have been suggested at the Department of Pathobiology of the University of Guelf, Canada [307]. They include (1) vaccine effectiveness with or without change of vaccine regimens, (2) vaccine delivery to middle-/low-income countries, (3) duration of immunity following vaccination, (4) vaccine hesitancy and long-term safety profile of COVID-19 vaccines, and (5) vaccine mistargeting. When twenty-three frail elderly individuals in Norway died shortly after receiving the Pfizer vaccine, the Scandinavian audience and the whole world was shocked. If many unpredicted severe long-term side-effects were to accrue over time, this could cause the withdrawal of approval for a vaccine. Another critical point is the effective duration of immunity of COVID-19 vaccines. From an epidemiological point of view, if immunity declines before "herd immunity" is achieved, previously vaccinated, individuals will become susceptible to infection again, and the rollout could fail or an iterative cycle takes place. Fragile effectiveness of COVID-19 vaccines relies on the lack of disclosure of Pfizer that there were large numbers of suspected but unconfirmed cases of COVID-19 that were excluded from their calculation of efficacy, reducing to 19-29%. The effectiveness reported for Sinovac Biotech's currently unapproved vaccine dropped from 78% to about 50%. Another point is the risk of variants that can evade vaccine-induced immunity. If some mutations promote the survival of SARS-CoV2 in vaccinated people, it could be disaster for the current strategy.

Vaccine hesitancy may have several roots, but one of the most intriguing would be the non-studied long-term safety profile of COVID-19 vaccines [301]. The recrudescence of measles in the most recent years is an important aspect to keep in mind. Measles (rubeola) is a highly contagious vaccine-preventable systemic disease caused by the measles virus, which belongs to the *Paramyxoviridae* family. The fever, runny nose, cough, and an enanthem (Koplik spots) precede an erythematous, maculopapular rash. It begins on the face and becomes more confluent as it spreads caudally. Complications have been recognized in 10% to 40% of patients, and treatment is predominantly symptomatic. Bacterial superinfections should be tackled with specific antibiotic therapy. Measles can be eradicated and needs to be eradicated because the complication rate approaches 1:2 cases. A universal childhood immunization and vaccination of all susceptible individuals with the measles vaccine is feasible. Humans are the only known hosts so far of measles. The virus is commonly transmitted by inhaling virus-laden airborne droplets or small-particle aerosols that may remain suspended in the air, direct contact with fomites, and infected secretions [51, 69]. It is important to recall that this microorganism can survive in the air or on fomites for up to 2 hours. Measles is a highly contagious systemic disease, which is often considered only cutaneous. It has been reported that up to 90% of susceptible contacts develop the disease [308]. Before introducing the vaccine, about nine children out of 10 contracted measles by the age of 15 years, but following the vaccine's introduction, measles became rare in North America and Europe, with most reported cases originating in Africa, Western Pacific, and South-East Asia. In North America, most cases are usually imported from countries where measles is endemic, but measles outbreaks may occur because of immunity gaps. In developed countries, vaccine negligence or refusal remains highly problematic and accountable for such outbreaks. It has been calculated that population vaccination rates must be over 93% if we need to eliminate measles. The current measles vaccines are live attenuated measles strains that replicate within the host to induce both humoral and cellular immunity. The first dose of the measles vaccine given at the age of 1-year protects well against the viral infection. The completion of vaccination results in 100% protection against measles. In the USA and Canada, routine immunization is recommended. Measles vaccines are generally safe and well-tolerated, but adverse effects can take place. They include fever, rash, and arthralgia and usually occur 5 to 12 days post-vaccination. There is a potential association between measles vaccine and acute disseminated encephalomyelitis (ADEM), which is an acute inflammation of both the cerebrum and spinal cord. The risk is not likely to be more than 1.16 cases of ADEM per million vaccines administered. Thus, the risk is extremely low, but the risk to die because of measles pneumonia is not trivial. Vaccine refusal and hesitancy have been invigorated in the last two decades due to misleading reports, unbalanced facts, and fake news circulating diffusely on social networks. One of the major accusations is the association between vaccine administration and autism. The accusation that the MMR vaccine may lead to autism spectrum disorders is substantially groundless [252]. The article awoke an enormous interest in both professional and lay outlets and forums, but unfortunately, it was fraudulent and deplorably retracted 12 years later. The major damage was the late retraction because the paper promoted parental concerns, turmoil in social and professional platforms, and skepticism on public-private partnerships about the safety of MMR vaccine, leading to lower vaccination levels and outbreaks of measles infection in several countries. One or two cases may raise a hypothesis, but data were missing to formulate a theory. A scrupulous evidence-based meta-analysis of five cohort studies (n=1 256 407) and five case-control studies (n=9920) found no evidence for a link between MMR vaccination and the subsequent development of autism or autistic spectrum disorders.

Credits and discredits have been associated with vaccines and vaccination on media coverage for decades. Polemics are jeopardizing some of the significant achievements in healthcare. Non-motivated vaccine hesitancy, delay, and vaccine refusal are continuously dominating healthcare front news with a dramatic increase of exanthemata in the last few years across the globe. Vaccine hesitancy may be due to safety concerns, low confidence in vaccines, and adequacy of specific recommendations. Physicians, parents, and anti-vaxxers cannot communicate correctly, and miscommunication has been amplified during the current COVID-19 pandemic. An increase of such preventable diseases in countries where these diseases seemed to be contained has characterized the headlines of both social media and professional platforms [253, 309, 310]. Our immune system's argumentation that can fight preventable diseases is affected by our children's relatively weaker immune response, different from the children of more than a hundred years ago. Family physicians are responsible for explaining to parents that vaccines benefit their children and other children, particularly by traveling in developing countries. COVID-19 disease, the infectious disease caused by SARS-CoV-2, is a pandemic that has reached all continents and caused numerous deaths worldwide, and the search for a vaccine is in progress [311]. The anti-vaxxers have populated many blogs and websites with diverse vaccine candidates, raising the shield against potential vaccines and recruiting several political figures at their rallies. The key is that several steps need to be reached before a vaccine can be distributed to the general population. Collective amnesia has permitted the increase of the anti-vaccine movement, whose careless followers believe vaccines are to line the pockets of Big Pharma. Amnesia involves the ignorance that the smallpox vaccine was so prodigiously successful at eradicating the disease that it no longer is habitually given. It has been estimated that the polio vaccine has saved 10 million people from paralysis only since 1988. It prevented 500,000 deaths, and a global vaccination campaign for measles that began in 2000 contained an expected 23 million deaths by 2018. In the United States and Canada, influenza season usually occurs in the winter. Numerous strategies are being explored to prevent the spread of influenza and minimize the risk of severe complications related to this infection. Influenza and COVID-19 infections may devastate our health care systems. If, during non-epidemic years, approximately 100,000 persons are admitted to the hospital due to influenza infection each year in the United States or Canada, the number of admissions to the hospital more than doubles during epidemic years [314]. Since the beginning of the tragic COVID-19 pandemic, the notion that people wearing face masks may protect themselves and others has been heavily politicized [69]. Anti-facemasks became the forerunners of the anti-SARS-CoV-2 vaccine protesters. The emphasis on individual freedom and distrust for institutional authority share a comparison to vaccines. Some people may have medical, mental health, or even communication issues that are legitimate reasons to be exempt from wearing masks. Still, most people should obey public health principles for the benefit of all communities [69]. Specific risk factors have been identified in University students with the tendency of believing in conspiracy theories in copying with stress [312, 313].

Social responsibility is a quest and should pervade our academic and non-professional environment. It is crucial to emphasize that vaccination is a personal choice and a question of social responsibility, international development, and institutional commitment that need to be expressed with integrity [301]. One of the ten risks to global public health is vaccine hesitancy [315]. Social responsibility is an ethical context where either an organization or an individual must act for the benefit of society. In the setting of individual social responsibility, it is mandatory to advocate political or social issues that can help others, e.g., advocating for policies targeting domestic and family violence in post-conflict communities. In this context, an egocentric view of choosing not to be vaccinated without consistent data should be considered irresponsible from a social point of view. In an international context, countries and societies have different degrees of development related to their pre-and post-colonial history, culture, and interaction with neighbors. The International Covenant on Economic, Social, and Cultural Rights (ICESCR) provides that all individuals are entitled to the gratification of the highest attainable standard of physical and mental health [316]. Our social commitment will be crucial in the 21st century in the framework of epidemics and the current pandemic. There will not be any victory for healthcare if dialog and empathy are not strengthened.

Conspiration and conspiration theories are two different things. Vaccine hesitancy and refusal may be associated with a legitimate desire to avoid foreign material inoculations, but conspiracy theories have propagated and emphasized. It is essential to remind that conspiration is one thing and conspiration theory is another. The Watergate was a conspiration, while the

5G-COVID-19 connection is a conspiration theory. The number of conspiracy theorists is increasing worldwide, and social media have put fuel on the fire. Although free speech is critical to be reminded of, the absence of a balance may jeopardize the health of ill and healthy children. QAnon is a conspiracy theory asserting that a secret cabal of Satan-worshipping, cannibalistic pedophiles run a global child sex trafficking ring. Diffuse pornography on the internet is on the rise and may target minors in some countries. Still, a massive conspiracy theory involving the entire globe and the current pandemic is insane. It leads to the destruction of the nation, making ground for foreign powers to take advantage of. QAnon and white supremacists risk jeopardizing the traditional republican values that they would like to defend. Substantially, the advantage of accepting any conspiracy theory may be damaging to the unity and solidity of the United States of America and Canada and the unwavering conservative values of Americans and Canadians. Acumen and perspicacity have been two essential characteristics of the traditional republican platform. There is no substantial and credible basis for such theories, apart from considering their pure research hypotheses. We need to remind that there is a well-standardized process of gathering data from idea to theory. The lack of data leads to a complete refusal of such conspiration theory. The scientific method, from a working hypothesis to a theory, entails well specific steps. However, even considering it from an operational view, a study design is challenging to implement. Thus, diffusing such rumors may increase people's anxiety, vaccine hesitancy, or refusal, and lead some groups ultimately to violence.

Chapter 10

Mass and Elite Cultures and Tolerance

Abstract

The need to shut down the phone is crucial to avoid an unstoppable increase in anxiety. But what is the difference in experiencing it seen by mass and elite cultures? Understanding these two cultures in our society is crucial, and the clash of the religions is nothing against the conflict of the cultures.

Keywords: culture, tolerance, Seneca, heritage

"*Quisquous*" and emphatic speeches can be deleterious. Why in some ages do we speak in a swollen way with mulled periods or with chant rhythm? Why are exaggerated translations used? Why is the oratory style affected by the variability of customs? If public eloquence is too lush, we face relaxation and decadence in our life. [*Quare quibusdam temporibus provenerit corrupti generis oratio quaeris, et quomodo in quaedam vitia inclinatio ingeniorum facta sit, ut aliquando inflata explicatio vigeret, aliquando infracta et in morem cantici ducta? Quare alias sensus audaces et fidem egressi placuerint, alias abruptae sententiae et suspiciosae, in quibus plus intellegendum esset quam audiendum? Quare aliqua aetas fuerit quae translationis iure uteretur inverecunde? Hoc quod audire vulgo soles, quod apud Graecos in proverbium cessit: talis hominibus fuit oratio qualis vita.*] These words would re-echo the current mass culture. These words of disapprovation are two millennia old. They are from Seneca's epistle to Lucilius. Seneca, a philosopher of the Roman Imperial Age, argues that pseudo-eloquence and not eloquence was permeating the culture. In particular, he pointed out three pseudo-eloquences present in his current age. Such deviation from the "true" eloquence can be seen currently as well. The education has been relegated to a kind of prostitute of politics defaming important equality principles. If we spend time teaching almost exclusively political principles, we will lose the education to have an open mind to understand politics. We risk having pseudo-analphabetism or frank illiteracy in future generations. Seneca suggested that pseudo-eloquence was seeping into his time. Some gross defect vitiates all three forms: the redundant and full of emphasis (*inflated*), the languid and stagnant, because it is made up of broken periods (*infracta*), and the one pronounced with singing voice (*in morem cantici ducta*), and therefore dull and artificial. In perusing the debates of the last political elections in several countries, the futile considerations between adversary factions inside the same cohorts, and the social platforms, it is easy to find some similarities with the defects Seneca suggested we are currently experiencing in our time. It is essential to raise the quality of our talk and not just forbid speeches. It is crucial raising words and not voices. Intellectual activities (*ingenium*) mirror the soul (*animus*). Some fundamental characteristics are specified: attitude, regularity, seriousness, balance, while sober vigor and moderation are highlighted in the intellectual activities. It is important to note that Seneca warns that the vice that spoils one also contaminates the other. It is important to maintain cultural competence using the intimate union between intellectual activity and soul preservation for eloquence. This cultural competence can be part of a core of democratic principles that can be taught, preserved, and screened to keep a "American or Canadian Citizenship" license. Each US citizen may be entitled to such a compulsory legal authorization every two years with core content involving Constitutional and Civil Law achievements and Anti-

Racism Laws in the United States and Canada, emphasizing the fights for freedom, which took place over the centuries worldwide. Thus, Holocaust, the Irish famine, India's independence battles, South Africa Mandela's Resistance, the Chinese Opioid Wars, the Tiananmen massacre, the Chinese cultural revolution, and the American and Canadian Residential Schools will be part of the information to keep the principles of democracy viable and vital in each citizen. Any extremism should and must be monitored.

Mass media have multiplied, and TV is now accompanied by Facebook, YouTube, Twitter, TikTok, and WeChat, among others. Pure, honest, and transparent eloquence is a missing tale of the current political puzzle. Looking at the situation and criticizing it about two millennia later is the late linguist and social and political commentator, Umberto Eco, an Italian medievalist, philosopher, semiotician, and fervid cultural critic. He is famous for some novels such as *The Name of the Rose* and *Foucault's Pendulum*. In his "*Apocalyptic and Integrated*" book, Eco presents an assembly of writings on the subject, which vary from socio-psychological studies of advertising and consumption to mass of industrial goods, to criticism on the intellectual's role individuals should undertake towards the mass media. In perusing the *Apocalyptic and Integrated* perceptions, it surfaces a Manichean attitude to either demonize media and cultural products inserted within the society of the image or praise and assimilate in the culture of origin. Eco's criticisms are crucial because the process of examining the political, economic, philosophical, and socio-political implications is often not thoroughly scrutinized. Several mass media have reduced the human being to a vilified individual who does not use intellectual activity anymore, and such contaminations have propagated to vitriolize the soul. It is the intimate connection of intellectual activity and soul, which is crucial for delivering eloquent speeches. However, to whom is a benefit "*cui bono*," we may consider pondering. The current degeneration is rampant and extremely worrying with aspects of a "*Bellum omnium contra omnes*" (i.e., "a war of everybody against everybody"). *Cui bono* expresses that crimes are often committed to benefit their offenders, especially financially, but a scapegoat may also be present. This scapegoat may be the constitution based on the principles of the Great Fathers. In the

"*Pro Roscio Amerino*" defense, Lucius Cassius, whom the Roman people regarded as a most honest and wise judge, was accused. Cicero argues in the habit of asking time "to whom might it be for a benefit?" [*L. Cassius ille, quem populus Romanus verissimum et sapientissimum iudicem putabat, identidem in causis quaerere solebat, cui bono fuisset?*] expressing the inadequacy of the crime sources [28, 29]. It is particularly crucial to ponder the concepts developed by the American sociologist Peter Blau, who used the idea of "*cui bono*" to differentiate organizations by who has primarily benefited: owners, members, or the general society. Facebook is the most extensively used social media platform in the Western world, with more than four-fifths of Canadians harboring an account. Facebook and other social media platforms do not produce original journalism but allow sharing news, either true or false or, if you like, legitimate or illegitimate. Facebook has taken an extreme step in reaction to an Australian law that would force Big Tech companies like Facebook and Google to pay media companies to use their content. As reported by the National Public Radio, an American privately and publicly funded non-profit media organization based in Washington, DC, the Information Commissioner's Office of the United Kingdom found that Facebook breached data protection laws. Facebook failed to keep users' personal information secure, allowing another company to gather the data of more than 80 million people without their consent worldwide [317].

Vision is key to saving humanity. There is an idea that conceives that the world is a reflex of the rationality of the Creator. It allows a remarkable bond between cosmology and anthropology. Wisdom, which builds matter and the world, is also essentially moral prudence, which gives directions to existence. The Torah (תּוֹרָה) is the Divine revelation to the humankind. Although commonly strictly considered the five books of Moses (Pentateuch), it can go to all the 24 books, from the Book of Genesis to the end of the Tanakh (Chronicles), and beyond. This conception approaches a conjunction from one side of Platonism or Neo-Platonism and to the other side of the stoic interpretation of the world and moral understanding. The concept of moral understanding is a crucial requirement for one's actions to be compatible with moral virtue. There are five principles, which are the cornerstone for ethical understanding [318]. The principles are autonomy, nonmaleficence, beneficence, loyalty, and justice. The abandonment of one of these principles may jeopardize our moral understanding. Also, such introspective exploration raises a better understanding of the conflicting issues of our society. Copernicus, Galilei, and Newton were platonic essentially. Their theses were based on the concept of the mathematical structure of the world. Their studies raise the importance to decrypt enigmas through experimentation. The tasks should be addressable, correctable, and utilizable. There is here the conjunction of Platonism and Empiricism. There is a flow from idea to experiment. If we limit our Reason, we will have a mutilated rationale. No free speech will mutilate our ability to express ourselves as human beings and this aspect is not understood in several intellectual and liberal circles. In reminding Descartes and its famous "*Cogito ergo sum* [I think, there I am/exist]," free speech and free thinking will leave us the freedom to think, the space to exist. We must ask ourselves about our origin and our end, and this eschatological journey will be determined by our ability to travel free with our minds. The syllogism (Socrates is a man, all men are mortal; therefore, Socrates is mortal) implies a conclusive sequence based on data (major and minor premises) validated. The combination of a general statement (the central premise) and a specific statement (the minor premise) leads to a conclusion or syllogism (συλλογισμός, 'inference'). Suppose we rely on to answer these questions to a belief, feeling or mere experience, i.e., separated from the Logos. In that case, we do not raise it to the highest level; we do not keep it solid but will remain fragile and subject to destruction. We dishonor these decisions if we do not apply the Logos. In the last few centuries, and mainly with Marxism and Nazism, the almost disintegration of man occurred. This disintegration starts when totalitarianism is permitted, when the economy flourishes, and technology advances. Such breakdown happens and destabilizes the health of both social sciences and science, but also religion. The Protocols of the Elders of Zion (Протоколы сионских мудрецов), alternatively known as the Protocols of the Meetings of the Learned Elders of Zion, is a fabricated antisemitic text purporting to describe a Jewish plan for global domination. First published in 1903, translated into multiple languages, and disseminated internationally in the early part of the 20th century, this literary forgery is probably the most influential work of antisemitism ever written. In reminding Wakefield's report and the vaccine hesitancy and refusal propagated, academia often notes that there is confusion between hypothesis and theory in non-scientific fields.

Hypothesis and theory are two different things. A fact is an introductory statement established by observation or experiment. Each "fact" is valid under specific conditions, but some facts may be false when re-tested with better instruments or observed at different conditions. For example, water boils at 212 Fahrenheit (100 degrees Celsius) is a fact, but close to Mount Everest, the water boils at a lower temperature. On the same level as fact is the belief, which is a statement that is not scientifically proved or testable. Beliefs can be facts, and scientifically disproven beliefs can still be held to be true. The hypothesis is a tentative statement, i.e., such as 'if A occurs, then B must happen' hypothesis that can be tested by observation or direct experiment. If the hypothesis is proven, it can be expressed as a theory or law. If the hypothesis is disproven, it can invalidate the statement and become a ground to re-test the information under different conditions or additional experiments. The theory is an explanation for why specific facts exist in nature, and these tentative statements or hypotheses are tested to determine their accuracy. Theories are usually based on a large body of proven hypotheses, although one tested hypothesis may trigger a theory. Also, a law is a logical relationship, which presupposes two conditions that need both to be accurate, including (1) a relationship between two or more entities, *and* (2) the relationship is based on a variety of facts and proven hypotheses.

Moral duty is critical in the pursuit of a scientific method. When we detach the Logos from the moral obligation or consider the moral responsibility as an abstract concept, we risk jeopardizing our human pathways. Euthanasia, human cloning, human experimentation, and other experiments can become readily accepted, but the negation of the Logos will destroy the individuum. At this time, science becomes pathologic and will inevitably destroy life. The science and the techniques used in the scientific methods become pathological and life-threatening when they leave the context of the moral order to humans. The importance of strict regulation on gene editing techniques, such as CRISPR-Cas9, cannot be emphasized enough. CRISPR-Cas9 is a technology that enables investigators to edit parts of the genome. We must go back to escape from our own "prison" we built ourselves after the French revolution and Modernism. Human forms of verification are fallible. We need something like what we find in Socrates: a personality with an ongoing availability maintained open and looked beyond itself. Degenerations are challenges to pursue higher aspirations. We live in a tetrad of degenerations, including degeneration of the language, costumes, morals, and memory with the erasing culture movements. In one passage of his works, Hegel, a philosopher of the 19th century, notes that all the significant facts of the history present themselves.

Culture needs to be refocused. We may consider focusing on some definition of culture and its intersection with society, politics, and religion. A culture is a form of expression of a community. Culture has a historical path, reaches a body of knowledge and is characterized by a solid judgment. Although this definition may be arduous to adapt to all niches of humankind, it may probably mirror the evolution of our understanding in terms of knowledge of culture. Of course, there are integrated and disintegrated degrees of culture that may characterize some aspects of our society. Culture is exclusively connected with knowledge values. Culture has, first, to do with knowledge values. It involves an attempt to understand the world and living man in it. It is a path guided by fundamental interests of our existence. Culture is not and should not be considered in individualistic terms. It is not linked to a man or woman mastering the world and life. It is essential to recognize that the world cannot be understood if we do not start a relationship with the Divine. This relationship was identified by the Founding Fathers when they enucleated the concept that culture was linked to justice for everyone. In terms of classicism, the culture includes the overcoming of the appearance of the visible world. The culture is connected to the Wisdom who stayed with the elderly and close to the Divinity. The primordial traditions have characters or features of the revelation. It is probably interesting to cite Giordano Bruno in agony between search and memory. The community is hugely linked to the investigative process. It proceeds progressively and is inextricably associated with a historiographic process. History is the study of the past, while historiography is the study of historical writing. Historiography is intriguingly linked to the development of a culture. The control of the historiographic process is paramount to avoid that only the winners are chosen to write history. Historiography is crucial for a wide range of reasons. First, it helps us understand why historical occurrences have sometimes been interpreted significantly differently over time. Historiography facilitates us to examine the history and the broader overlying attributes that shape the exact recording of history itself. Historiography is never politically correct, but history or historical writing may run on this road according to the evolution of the culture. The unique expertise is crucial in transforming the culture and identifying the different channels for dialogue. It is not an easy process because the discussion may annihilate or be re-dimensioned in monologue. The conversation is critical for the dynamics of the integration of the cultures. It is vital to the relationship with the Divine because a proper search starts with the humble request in identifying ways of dialogue. The egocentricity and narcissism of cultures or individuals may become self-destructive. Thus, historiography comes back as a crucial aspect and amalgam for the investigative process of the culture.

Tolerance is the response to save humanity. Our minuscule effort to clarify the fundamental categories of the conceptualization of culture derives from our prerequisite that it will help us better understand the different possibilities of contact and fusion between cultures. This approach is key to focusing on the link of a culture to a cultural individuality, to a specific subject that assembles the diversity of cultures considering their specificity and particularity. Memory is necessary, which relies on experience. The term experience arises from Latin, and it includes the process (dynamic, not static) of useful contact with and careful observation of facts or events. The different cultures meet with cultural objects and must be compared with the inherent experiences. Thus, we must consider the culture's openness is crucial for the learning process of culture. The culture needs to acquire facts or events and can communicate with other cultures. It is now essential to record the tolerance present at the time of the Roman culture from the origins and extended to the maximal extension of the Adrian Empire. We often encountered in history books a period called "*Pax Romana*." This period, which translates to "Roman peace," refers to the time from 27 BC to 180 AD during the Roman Empire. The about two centuries period saw unprecedented peace and economic prosperity throughout the Roman Empire. It was a period often considered felicitous for numerous generations. The empire extended from England in North Europe to Morocco in South Europe and from Brittany and Aquitaine in West Europe to Mesopotamia in the East within the Tigris–Euphrates river system. Mesopotamia corresponds with Iraq, Kuwait, the eastern parts of Syria, Southeastern Turkey, and areas along the Turkish–Syrian and Iran–Iraq borders. The success of the Roman Empire established that the Romans had a regular and systematic worshipping. The Romans were strongly tolerant of other peoples' divinities, allowing natives in their provinces to worship their divinities unless they were bringing political or social unrest. However, there was also something special in the Roman society. Racism was not a characteristic of the society. Slaves, yes, but racism not. Our consideration of slaves reconnects to the Black community transferred from Africa to England, France, and United States. The concept of slaves in Roman Antiquity was different. It is essential to ponder notes of priests and monks visiting Africa, converting black communities from animistic spirituality to Christianity. While slavery was a deeply stigmatized social status, most slaves were from Mediterranean and European populations. Also, inherited physical characteristics were not relevant to slave status. Black people were not excluded from any profession in Rome. Furthermore, there was usually no stigma or bias against mixed-race relationships in Antiquity. There are some good examples. A centurion with the name of Vocusius Africanus is documented from Vindolanda on Hadrian's Wall, and prominent Romans with origins in North Africa include Lucius Quietus, a Moorish officer under Trajan, and even the Emperor Septimius Severus, born in Lepcis Magna. Thus, the appropriation of the Roman Antiquity by white supremacists has no historical background.

Neutrality in science is complex and has been challenging during this pandemic, as future generations will prove.In many cases, political calculus went over ideological concepts. Unfortunately, the neutrality of science for politics has been compromised, and a number of editorials have been published to support the current US administration indicating baseless attacks on the former US administration [319-329]. Is this the dialogue that science would like to encourage when more than seventy million voters supported the previous administration? Such vitriol attacks may jeopardize reconciliation in any country. It is important to remind that science is evolving. The concepts used at the beginning of the pandemic from the CDC have been identified as not wholly correct and rectified later. The difficulty of non-scientists in dealing with science matters makes them fragile and prone to error and scrutiny because they do not have the full picture. Thus, caution should be the next step in leading biomedical journals or social platforms where they ostracize the opponents. The importance of a balance in platforms supporting dialogues is crucial in the 21st century [330]. A contentious new rule of the European Union (EU) on copyright says that news aggregators and search engines should pay news websites for links. There have been other topics of tension between governments and Big-Tech companies, where governments or unions such as the EU have investigated regulating the firms in question. The polarization of the recent US elections may call for the regulation of this sector. Almost in all periods of Ancient Greek literature, *μῦθος* and *λόγος* co-exist but have two distinct meanings. Indeed, Mythos (*μῦθος*) relies upon narrative and informal knowledge. At the same time, Logos (*λόγος*) refers to logical and rational analysis of the phenomena. It has been described that their interaction creates various forms with variable predominance. Thus, the boundaries between them are not strictly fixed [331]. We see in current politics an abnormality in the equation "*qualis vita, talis oratio*." Between πόλις and ποίησις, it is important to differentiate. While πόλις refers to a city, but also self-governance, independence, and autonomy (city-state), the word ποίησις entails "the activity in which a person brings something into being that did not exist before" [332]. Solon of Athens, an Athenian statesman, powerful lawmaker, and delicate poet of Ancient Greece, is the memory of posterity because of his efforts to legislate against the political, economic, and moral decline in archaic Athens. According to the Athens' Constitution, Solon legislated for all citizens to be admitted into the assembly (ἐκκλησία). A vital court (Ἡλιαία) was created to be formed from all the citizens. Thus, Solon is probably correctly credited with having laid the foundations for democracy in Athens and posterity. His learning avidity was insatiable. In the Florilegium, Stobaeus relates a story about a symposium where Solon's young nephew sang Sappho's poem. In his senility, Solon was asked why to bother learning a skill at his age, and he replied, "ἵνα μαθὼν αὐτὸ ἀποθάνω," "So that I may learn it before I die." [333]. The importance of education is mirrored from these fulgid examples that need to revive our souls, avoiding glazing screens of smartphones for hours each day. Solon is probably the first to explain the connection between literary work (ἔργον) and rational (λόγος). Solon reported in Diogenes Laertius I.58 is used to say that the λόγος – our "*oratio*," our speech – is an image (εἴδωλον) of our work or action (ἔργον) [334]. Demosthenes claimed that Athens' subsequent golden age included "personal modesty and frugality" among the Athenian aristocracy. Demosthenes and posterior critics consider that Solon, by both personal example and legislated reform, established an absoluteprecedent for this decorum in Antiquity.

Chapter 11

SOLIDARITY, SOCIAL, AND SOCIALISM

ABSTRACT

This chapter presents roots and pathways for humanity to recover from the pandemic. We dare to criticize ourselves to improve and rejuvenate the social contract between rulers and citizens.

Keywords: wisdom, humanity, society, socialism, social capitalism.

Humanity is nowadawy confused, but it is not the first time in history. We are at the crossroads and we may need to remember Hildegard von Bingen's words to search for directions. *Wie sich die beiden Hände, wenn sie ans Werk gehen, miteinander vereinigen und wie auch Himmel und Erde, so sehr sie sich unterscheiden mögen, in einer gewissen Gemeinschaft zusammenstehen, so vollendet auch der Mensch durch die verschiedenen Wissensmöglichkeiten, die er besitzt, jede Handlung* (Just as the two hands unite with each other when they go to work and just as heaven and earth, however different they may be, stand together in a certain community, so too does the human being complete every action through the various possibilities of knowledge that he possesses) [297]. In any century there are few people who have a peculiar character and pregnant personality. Their words and deeds have shaped not only their generation but also the future generations. The words and deeds of wise women and men have given decisive important impulses to the society and humanity. The Abbess Hildegard von Bingen (1098-1179) is such a person and shaped an important generation of the 12th century. Her words of wisdom, inspiration, and reassurance have been pillar for powerful and famous people, but also for simple families and farmers who constantly visited her abbey. Her attitude to dialogue with both high and low levels of the society in a decent manner is key to understand her influential personality. Also, she used her illness to understand the soul better. Hildegard von Bingen had a special relationship with both the Lord and humans. She sanctified each day with words and actions of remarkable wisdom. She had a pharmaceutical herb garden in her monastery and an astonishing knowledge of the processes occurring in nature. Songs and hymns originate in her monastery. In wonderful pictures and beautiful language, the glory of the created world is portrayed to celebrate the unity of Heaven and Earth. The primeval climate activist noted that everything depends on everything together. Nothing can be viewed in isolation. In consideration of Hildegard von Bingen's words, we still need to have a plea for unity everyday. Both democratics and republicans in the United States of America and liberals and conservartives in Canada must plea for unity and avoid squandering the wisdom acquired in centuries of unity of the countries. In writing from prison in Rome, Paul underlines that to partake with him is important to defend and confirm. In the Ἀπολογία (Apology) there is the defense or answer of a text or an action, but βεβαίωσις (Confirmation) entails the validation. A defense alone is not often enough to let the counterpart accepting the apology. It is crucial a confirmation of the apology. This attitude no matter from which part arises should always be perfused in our speeches and deeds. Both components anchor and consolidate the bridge for collaboration. There is an untold story that a man had to prepare himself to govern his kingdom and went to visit three wise men in an old mountain where no roads were marked. He was advised that this path had to enterpreun on his own. In the early morning, he approached the three men subsequently. The first wise man tells the future kind "Your enemies are those in front to recognize right away", while second wise man inspires him indicating that his enemies are his friends, substantially those that he could not easily recognize. The third man shocked him because he told him "Your worst enemy is your self because it is the Troy's horse within your soul". The tale is that while the first pathway was easy to find and the second was ambiguous, the third one was the most challenging, because was concealed and mischievous. We see perennial life cursed by drink, brutality and vice, and loaded down with ignorance and poverty, while education is still painfully mounting and slipping back from our original path as magnificently indicated by Charles Booth, a British shipping magnate in 1903 [335].

1848 was a year characterized by various turbulence in Europe. There were uprisings in Italy (Sicily, Naples, Rome, Florence, Tuscany, Piedmont, Venice, Milan), Germany (Baden, Wurttemberg, Nassau, Hesse-Darmstadt, Bavaria, Saxony), France, Denmark, Belgium, Holland, Prussia, Austria, Hungary, Czech, Ireland, Great Britain, and Sweden. 1848 is additionally the year the Communist Manifesto is published. Although examples of communities sharing their wealth have been recorded in human history, this landmark represents the proper exposure of the Western world to communist views. Marx and Engels indicated the uneven distribution of wealth in the capitalist world. The authors aimed to redistribute wealth evenly. Some countries had incorporated this view in governments with failure or inadequate final goals. The damage of communism has been devastating, and millions of people died and continue to die in countries where communism is applied. The USSR or Union of the Soviet Socialist Republics existed from 1922 to 1991. The USSR embraced the politics that the government and economy must be exclusively centralized. During the USSR and the Cold War with the USA, genocides were perpetrated and periods of famine occurred. In any communist country, no matter how much capital is introduced to keep the philosophy of communism alive, there is also a lack of freedom and free choice. The danger is that the human being may embrace this form of government as long bread is on the table.

The ideology of the Chinese Communist Party (CCP) has dramatically developed since Mao Zedong and is continuously reassessing with the world economy. Some authors state that the CCP currently lacks a coherent ideology, while others indicate that the CCP still identifies itself as a communist party. Historically and practically speaking, the current CCP is quite different from the original CCP. The wealth, the technology, the progress, and the education reached in most of the provinces are great, potentially at the expense of freedom. The CCP now allows its citizens to keep some or most of the profits they earn comparable to Western democracies standards. Beijing has also an incredible number of billionaires. Uncommitted behavior has been identified as the culprit for the initial failure of the communist ideology, particularly in the article "Revolutionary Ideals are Higher than Heaven-Studying" [336]. The author writing under the pen name "Autumn Stone," supports the current CCP General Secretary policy of strengthening the ideological conviction in the CCP and the party cadres. The ideology advocates eliminating any opponent or lightly diverging opinion. The author suggests that such ideological unity leads to party unity. Also, uncommitted ideals and convictions are considered to represent the most harmful indecisiveness that may lead to dissolution. Thus, reading this article and carefully studying the data related to the current effects of policies makes it clear that freedom of expression seems to be quite far in China. Several articles and reports outside of China are considered unimaginable in mainland China. In the cited article above, the word corruption is assigned to people who have uncommitted ideals. It claims that the dissolution of the Soviet Union was linked to officials' hesitancy, citing that even Mikhail Gorbachev, the last USSR leader, had acknowledged that communist ideals had become antediluvian to him.

Leviathan is a book penned by Thomas Hobbes (1588–1679) during the English Civil War (1642–1651) and published in 1651 with translations in numerous languages [337]. In his book, the author deals with the structure of society and legitimate government. It is probably one of the earliest and most prominent examples of social contract theory. Hobbes supports a social contract and the rule by an absolute sovereign following the economic and human disaster of the English Civil War. His consideration is1 supported by the Latin proverb of "*Homo homini lupus*," which means that a man is a wolf to another man. This sentence derives from the play "Asinaria" in 212 BC by Plautus: "*Lupus est homo homini, non homo, quom qualis sit non novit*" emphasizing the hostility present in the human beings [338]. There is, indeed, the brute and ghastlycircumstances of a state of nature ("*Bellum omnium contra omnes*" or "the war of all against all") in Hobbes' scared memory. The English Civil War may have some similarities to the Western Imperialistic domination or Opium Wars against China and, partly, to the Japanese invasion of China before WWII. The sufferences of the Chinese people are rarely mentioned in the Western culture and this is not fair. Overall, this state of nature and brutality could be avoided only by a strong, fully committed, and undivided government. In Hobbes' book, the commonwealth is instituted when all agree to authorize and give up the right of governing to the government chief. Totalitarianism imposes a form of government where the authority uses absolute and centralized control over all of the most relevant aspects of life. The individual is subordinated to the state. Any opposition or political and cultural expression is carefully controlled or suppressed. Hobbes identifies some principal rights in the ruler's figure due to a covenant between citizen and ruler. They include 1) the impossibility to change the form of government, 2) the solidity of the commonwealth based on the impossibility to breach the covenant, 3) the complete abide of the minority if any to the arrangements set by the ruler and the majority, 4) the invalidity of any injustice accusation because every subject is author of the acts of the sovereign, 5) the authority has, substantially, the full power to do whatever is considered necessary for preserving peace and security, and prevention any kind of discord. No evident opposition is allowed. In consequence of it, the ruler magistrates what opinions and doctrines are opposed to the commonwealth. Under this principle, the ruler and majority will allow those who may speak to multitudes. A thorough examination of any work is emphasized before it is published. Also, the ruler prescribes civil law and property rules, judging in all cases that may be adverse to the ruler and majority. Hobbes explicitly rejects the idea of the Separation of Powers and favors censorship of the press and restrictions on the rights of free speech to promote order and harmony. In a nutshell, any totalitarian regime is inextricably linked to Hobbes' work. In this book, Hobbes coined the expression "*auctoritas non veritas facit legem*," which means "authority, not truth, makes law."

Socialism and communism allow the ruler to command. In socialism, like communism, there is a significant call for putting the major means of production in the hands of the people. Socialists believe in the redistribution of wealth in a softer way than communists, but in the end, there is redistribution. The aim is to reduce the gap between the rich and the poor and substantially confiscate or gather other people's wealth either using high taxes or promulgating restrictive laws. The centralized view and centralized power are present in both communism and socialism. They are substantially unchanged, but divergent opinions in socialism are often not manifestly crushed. Currently, there is not a purely capitalist or communist economy in the world. There is the need to sustain layers of society that need financial support. The capitalist-based United States of America has a Social Security system and a government-owned postal service. These agencies are just a few of the numerous benefits for the disadvantaged people that are linked to the government [339]. Canada has a similar system, but the higher level oftaxes allows a more considerable redistribution of wealth. The risk of the socialism is mirrored in the history and is linked to growing inactivity when the workers can receive income without work. The Canadian Recovery Benefit has been abused during the current pandemic. There is a risk that Canada and some Western democracies may be on the route to becoming socialistic countries *de facto* following the introduction of an universal basic income.

Social capitalism or "mild" capitalism has been suggested. It may harbor the principle of capitalism, which is respected. There is private proprietorship of the means of production and individual economic freedom. Most of the means of production are owned by private individuals and not nationalized by the government. Free competition and supply and demand are critical for capitalistic societies. In social capitalism, the ideology of liberty, equality, and justice is linked to capitalism's basic principles. However, instead of aiming for wealth redistribution or universal basic income, social capitalism explicitly values all forms of capital, and not only the economic forms. It adds a human factor and the promotion of wealth and health with the inspiration of any individual to pursuit happiness. Natural capital, social capital, and human capital are inextricably connected.

Solidarity is an essential aspect of the living community. Recently, a shocking COVID-19 patient portrait was published [340]. Stories like that have been surfacing in social networks for months. We need to reawaken ourselves and embolden social aspects in any act of life. The solidarity surcharge or Solidaritätszuschlag (SolZG or colloquially known as "Soli") has been a key supplement income to the income and corporation tax in Germany. The fall of the Berlin wall together with the subsequent reunification of East Germany to West Germany were economically challenging events for post-WWII Germany. Initially limited to one year in 1991, this surcharge has now been in place for almost three decades. Since 1998 the toll targeted 5.5% of income and corporation tax (§4 SolzG) [341]. According to German law, the federal government alone is entitled to the revenue and does not require the approval of the Bundesrat. In 2018, the revenue amounted to 18.93 billion euros. Although considered at least initially to cover the costs of the 2nd Gulf War (Jan-Mar 1991) and some Southern European countries, the surcharge was substantially justified to support the reconstruction of German unity. Primarily, the costs were devoted to the rebuilding of East Germany after the economic failure of this part of the country. The German Democratic Republic (Deutsche Demokratische Republik, DDR) was a country that existed from 1949 to 1990. This time corresponds to the eastern portion of Germany being part of the Eastern Bloc during the Cold War (1947-1991). This period mirrors the geopolitical tension between the USSR and the USA and their respective allies after WWII, spanning from the Truman Doctrine to the 1991 dissolution of the Soviet Union. Some quotes from the federal office of political education stated that 'In 1991 alone, 153 billion Deutschmarks had to be transferred to eastern Germany to secure incomes, support businesses and improve infrastructure... by 1999 the total had amounted to 1.634 trillion Deutsche Marks. This amount is equivalent to 1,011,563,718,512.46 or about one trillion US dollars, and one trillion is 10^{12}, and one EUR is equivalent to 1.95583 Deutsche Marks. Substantially, the sums were so large that public debt in Germany more than doubled' [342]. The three major political parties forming the government were key in relieving significantly lower and middle incomes from the solidarity surcharge. The two liberal conservatives CDU (or Christian Democratic Union of Germany) and CSU (or Christian Social Union of Bavaria) joined the SPD (or Social Democratic Party of Germany) in finding commonalities in the political sphere of the post-WWII era. Although the constitutionality of the solidarity surcharge has been challenged for many years, tax court judgments have been controversial. On February 11th, 2008, the Federal Constitutional Court did not accept the constitutional complaint. On September 8th, 2010, the Federal Constitutional Court ruled that additional taxes are not limited in time. Despite discussion about abolition for years, in 2019, there were plans that single employees would only have to pay the surcharge from 2021 onwards with a gross annual income of more than € 74,000. The Federal Audit Office advocates the complete abolition of the SolZG by the end of the new financial planning period in 2023 at the latest.

Domination of one's resentments is not an easy task during any catastrophic event. On April 28th, 1955, a global event took place in Athens, Greece, with the utopic aim of creating a Europe without internal borders and sentiments waved turbulently ten years after WWII. Albert Camus (1913–1960), novelist, philosopher, and essayist, born in Algeria from a Spanish mother and a Breton father, said that the wounds of the war had just ended [343]. These wounds were too fresh for everybody to hope that national collectives would make the utopia a reality, but only "superior" individuals would be capable. This superiority was neither class-related nor lineage- nor wealthy-related but consisted in overcoming their resentments in the events of catastrophes. Remarkably, an atheist and Marxist was formulating tones of reconciliation in his talk. Reading his works, mostly "The Stranger" and "The Plague," it is easy to enucleate Christian messages, probably more merciful than other professed Christians sitting there at that time. Camus was an active member of the anti-Nazi resistance and was awarded the Nobel Prize for literature in 1957 [344-347]. Camus was a Marxist, but he often found incoherence in the Communist Party. He eventually left the party [343]. Camus understood that the law might serve to divide the world between those who apply it and those who suffer it. He suggested that the moral laws are within each of us. Camus fundamentally emphasized the importance of the ability to master one's resentments to reach harmony. Dominating one's grievances is not an easy task during a pandemic. Social media and TV networks are vitrioling our souls against each other. We need to come back to the roots of the original Christian message of love, solidarity, compassion, respect, and mercy, no matter the skin color or the wealth of the status. We need to come together. Governments of national unity are in extreme need. It has been great that most of the United States presidents have been Lord-fearing men, who almost all have professed belief in the Sacred Books, and none was atheist. Presumably, the Divine Presence led the Great Founders of America and Canada. Although some signs of post-modernism, wild liberalism, social media deterioration are abounding. They are wildly running all over the nations. Still, there is hope that the Lord protects the United States of America and Canada. Yet, we need to pray for unity and solidarity among factions and parties. The leaders' prayer is crucial for any Christian to let them lead quietly, efficiently, and effectively.

Chapter 12

American Dream

Abstract

In this chapter, we present an introspection and reflection of the Pandemic. In the pandemic, as in the cholera of Gabriel Garcia Marquez, true love is undeniable and true love brings hopes in despair. The love for the American Dream is vital for the future of the World. Searching the roots, preserving them, and outgrowing them will develop paths to find hopes in despair in the time of pandemic and beyond.

Keywords: American, dream, politics, future

Let me tell you something you already know. The world ain't all sunshine and rainbows. It's a very mean and nasty place, and I don't care how tough you are it will beat you to your knees and keep you there permanently if you let it. You, me, or nobody is gonna hit as hard as life. But it ain't about how hard ya hit. It's about how hard you can get hit and keep moving forward. How much you can take and keep moving forward. That's how winning is done! Now, if you know what you're worth, then go out and get what you're worth. But ya gotta be willing to take the hits, and not pointing fingers saying you ain't where you wanna be because of him, or her, or anybody! Cowards do that, and that ain't you! You're better than that! This inspirational statement is probably one of the most lovely acts Sylvester Stallone, the fictional boxer, could give not only to his nation but to humanity [348]. It is expressive, passionate, painful, and inspirational. It is paramount to understand the American Dream no matter which political party the individual belongs to.

Communism and Socialism are a disgrace to humanity and well-being. Currently, it has been argued that some Western countries are more socialist than China, and if we leave America and Canada, our magnificent countries, to liberal progressives, the fate will be the same. The American dream will eventually end, because Canada is historically bound to the United States of America [349]. Both communism and socialism are ideologies that have caused deaths and poverty, similar to Nazism and Fascism. The number of victims of all four political systems is outrageous to humanity. It stands disgraceful when the Evangelion is reported in the wrong way. The Catholic Church has been wrongly considered an "*ante literam*" communism, but it is improper. Often proposed by some Fathers of the Liberation of Latin America, the Catholic Church should not be seen as an example of communism. In the religious Acts of the Apostles, it is indicated that 'no one considered his property what belonged to him or her, but between them everything was common.' It is not communism, but it is pure Christianity. Sharing one's possessions is not communism [350]. Any time the Communists took power, they shared each other's property. They redistribute wealth by claiming to abolish private property in the name of state property, and they make the dominion of the Communist Party. In the Acts, there is a free and voluntary choice of the faithful. Moreover, it is a religious community, not the State, and indeed Jesus Christ invites us to distinguish between Caesar (State) and God (Religion). Third, historians know that such redistribution of goods produced disagreements and resentments in the Christian community with a morally unsuccessful outcome. The experiment leads the Christians of Antioch (Acts 11:29) and then the Apostle Paul himself (2 Cor) to make collections for the brothers who had ended up in serious difficulties (Romans 15.26-27). Socci and numerous theologists indicated that instead of selling their properties and donating the proceeds to the community for the poor, they had made them an income. Giving part for charity would have done well to their community without reducing themselves into poverty. It is not possible to distribute wealth if we do not produce it.

Words have consequences because no one has the maturity to understand the boundaries of Reason. Independent from the appalling and horrifying events of the riots of January 6th, 2021, against the Capitol, let us know how words can exasperate and desperate people. There is no doubt that it was an attack on democracy, but any people committed to acting may exhibit distress. The analysis of the events with calm and cautious objectivity over subjectivity suggests stress, exasperation, and desperation. Inspirational videos cried an alarm toward the American people to stop listening to the media [351, 352]. We must use the brain again to address objectivity and reject allegations no matter where they come from without data that corroborates their veridicality. It is at this time that we recall Giordano Bruno's alarm (*... because truth is the most sincere, most divine thing of all: indeed Divinity is sincerity, goodness and beauty of things and truth; which is neither removed by violence, nor by antiquity it is corrupted, nor by occultation it is diminished, nor by communication it is dispersed: because sense does not confuse it, time does not ruin it, place does not hide it, night does not interrupt it, darkness does not hold it: on the contrary, with being more and more challenged, the more and more it resurrects and grows; without defender and protector she defends herself, and yet she loves the company of a few and wise men, she hates the multitude, she does not show herself to those who do not seek it for themselves, and does not want to be declared to those who humbly do not expose themselves to all those who fraudulently inquire it: and yet she dwells very high where all look, but few see* "perché la verità è la cosa piu sincera, piu divina di tutte: anzi la divinita e la sincerita, bonta e bellezza de le cose e la verità; la quale ne per violenza si toglie, ne per antiquita si corrompe, ne per occultazione si sminuisce, ne per communicazione si disperde: perche senso non la confonde, tempo non l' arruga, luogo non l' asconde, notte non l'interrompe, tenebra non l'avela: anzi con essere piu e piu impugnata, piu e piu risuscita e cresce; senza difensore e protettore si defende, e pero ama la compagnia di pochi e sapienti, odia la moltitudine, non si dimostra a quelli che per se stessa non la cercano, e non vuol essere dechiarata a color che umilmente non se gli esponeno, ne a tutti quei che con frode la inquireno: e pero dimora altissima dove tutti remirano, e pochi veggono") [353]. Ben Carson faced death many times when working as a neurosurgeon, a profession very similar to the pathologist who meets suffering and dying every day. Ben Carson's words are important because our mind is easy to manipulate. We need to remain focused recollect that other countries may have some better system, but the United States of America is unique. We can make mistakes and experience failures, but the freedom and the opportunities present in the American Dream are individual and are not present in any other country of this world. On the other hand, we need to be very careful in choosing words either with friends or crowds. We have a legacy with our Ancestors, and this legacy is vivid as long we discover and keep our roots in the text of the Constitution.

Education is a critical cornerstone in our society and is the lymph nourishing the organs of our community. Education needs hard commitments from both teachers and students. Creativity is the powerful force behind the most significant ideas, the most comprehensive solutions, and the profitable enterprises. The future of humanity depends on imaginative, creative, innovative solutions to thoughtful and complex challenges. There is more to say about Bruno's beautiful pages dedicated to the praise of Fatigue in the 3rd dialogue of the Dealership of the triumphant beast. The modern hedonistic pedagogy that inspired the recent school reforms of post-modernism should be considered irreverent and frightening to human thought. They are strikingly perseverating in the university, reducing the option of free speech to a minimal field of action. Lowering the level of education, making everything more accessible, does not help train new youth generations. In the texts, there is the passion that knowledge is not a gift but a tiring achievement. Teaching a child to read and loves reading and books is crucial and extremely important when youth constantly glazes their smartphones, even during Valentine's day dinners. However, there is more to comment on how actual knowledge can only result from free love for Wisdom and Reason. Bruno was a Copernican adept similar to Galilei, but his detachment from the Ptolemaic system, also called the geocentric system or geocentric model, was associated with Egyptian features of astronomy, probably less astronomical and more philosophical. The geocentric model of the universe formulated by the astronomer and mathematician Ptolemy about 150 AD was the thesis adopted by the Catholic Church. The Vatican condemned Giordano Bruno in 1600 and Galileo Galilei, thirty-three years later, for their putatively subversive views. On October 31st, 1992, the catholic Pope John Paul II formally apologized for the perseverance in the geocentric model. It was the first of some famous apologies during his papacy. Nobody is over the Reason, and science is full of truths that may be challenged, but they need to be understood and thought correctly. The Einstein relativity theory surpasses the Newton or Euclidian physics conceptsbut does not deny its use until quantum theory concepts are assimilated. The love for the wisdom and knowledge (φῐλόσοφος from φῐ́λος or "love" and σοφός or "skilled with handcrafts, wise, study") is crucial and needs to be taught with science during the years of formation. The word philosophy is defined as "the love of wisdom." It is studying the fundamental and profound matters of human existence and applying our human existence to the surrounding world and transcendence.

Confederates' belief was wrong in perpetuating an inhuman condition for human people. Although some may have some affection for the confederates, we need to recognize that it is still painful to watch confederate flags in American houses or buildings. It is not disputable that freedom is present, but we need to recognize that slavery was evil and not red-flagged and ostracized properly during the last four or five decades. It is not about erasing culture. It is re-appropriate and re-size the influences of the parties. It is respect toward the Black and Latino communities as well as other minorities. At times I was meat-eater and not particularly church observant. I always considered Paul's preaching, letters, and teaching. It is important to avoid eating disorderly, avoiding eating forbidden food in front of people who may feel disgusted seeing us eating such animals. If we go back to the roots of the two millennia of history, we re-discover that the respect of other religions, creeds, beliefs, and skin color is crucial for the solidity of this nation. The heritage of slavery and the damage will be part of our human history, similar to the Jewish Holocaust perpetrated by Nazi Germans. If we remember and teach these events without hate, we will discover human failure and re-discover the Divinity. The fraternity, which is highly promulgated by several constitutions, cannot be arid. The Reason made the Fathers of the American Costitution invoking God in the first three words ("We the People"). This call is for everyone to understand that our roots are a Divine sacrifice. There is no doubt that Black Africans kidnapped and transferred as merchandise from Africa to Europe or America was an evil act, and this started in a Christian country. Afonso I (1460-1542), also known as Mvemba a Nzinga, was the ruler of Kongo. It was the king of a powerful and historical kingdom in west-central Africa [354]. He was the first of a line of Portuguese kings that lasted until the early 20th century. In Africa, but elsewhere, he is called "*The Apostle of Kongo*" for his crucial role in making Kongo a Christian kingdom [355]. He exchanged an extraordinary series of letters with several kings and government officials in Rome and Lisbon. In 1491, Portuguese priests baptized him and his father, who assumed Christian names. After defeating his half-brother in battle, he succeeded as the king at the beginning of the 16th century, becoming the sixth king of the Kongo). According to his own account, his army started praying, more fervidly and appealed to St. James for assistance. St. James appeared in the sky along with five sworders, and the vision frightened the pagans, who abandoned the field [355]. During his reign, Afonso extended Kongo's relations with Portugal by accepting Portuguese institutions, granting extraterritorial rights to Europeans, mainly from Portugal, and supplied criminals to Portuguese traders. This part is probably crucial for understanding later slavery as an evil act. His faith was true, and being portrayed as Constantine of Africa may not be an exaggeration. He worked to introduce the Catholic religion in West Africa by demolishing traditional paganism and animism. His sincere acts of faith were inside of his family and his citizens. Apart from commemorations of the feast of St. James, a national holiday, and recognized Catholicism as the state religion of the Kongo, he encouraged the founding of confraternities and missionary schools that instructed the Congolese in Christian doctrine. Although the ordainment of his son as a bishop by Pope Leo X may be considered tactical, his attachment to the Christian faith was genuine, and it perspires in his letters denouncing the kidnapping and merchandise of free Congolese by Europeans. The Apostle of Congo's invective against slavery reached an acme when he discovers in 1526 that Portuguese merchants were purchasing illegally enslaved persons and exporting them. It is controversially debated how much Christian belief was present in Afonso's Congolese citizens, but this is often also questioned for Constantine and the first Roman Christian communities. Any leader who moves the political weight behind the Church may be questioned, but there are passionate letters, and the struggle present in these letters suggests he was experiencing evil acts under his own eyes. In one of such epistles, the sincerity of Afonso's faith was evident because he was willing to hold to its precepts and doctrine even as relations with Portugal deteriorated. Slaves were indeed present in Ancient times, but they consisted mainly of criminals and prisoners of war. These slaves were condemned to serve in aristocratic households or produce for cheap labor. There was a growth of an international market for slaves, mainly Europe and then America. The profit generated was massive. It pushed many Europeans and Congolese away from a low-key domestic model toward a florid but criminal economy based on greed. The words in Afonso's epistles show the sufferance of a king and the greed of merchandise. "Each day, the traders are abducting our people … This venality and depravity are so common that our land is entirely deserted. …The lure of profit and greed led people to rob their compatriots, including members of their own families." It is hard to discern between the defense of his kingdom against pagan relatives or the defense of his kingdom against a Christian foreigner. However, there is surmounting hypocritical greed of both Christian traders and some Congolese complices. He is aware of how the heartbreaking selfishness of his people may destroy the country. There is also a consistent text in his correspondence and fidelity to Lord's law independently from gold or gifts he may have received. His death, in 1542, signs the unbearable pain of a man who stood unwavering for his faith. After that, it has been estimated that some 10-12 million Africans were brought into America across the Atlantic in chains. Many of them died along the way. We need to stay together in front of this tragedy because all lives matter, even that of our perpetrator. There is a movement to come back to the roots. This aspect will involve the instauration of our Fathers' philosophy and social and human capital, which allows the re-vivification of the American dream keeping the Lord in and the whole nation in our prayers, and supporting respect for everyone, the People.

Change is key even in the preservation of traditional values. In a nutshell, we can recall the words of Viktor E. Frankl "When we are no longer able to change a situation – we are challenged to change ourselves" [356]. The book's original title in German is "*...trotzdem Ja zum Leben sagen: Ein Psychologe erlebt das Konzentrationslager*." (...Nevertheless saying Yes to Life: A Psychologist Experiences the Concentration Camp). This book was listed last century as one of the ten most influential books in the States by the Library of Congress [357]. Viktor E. Frankl (1905-1997) was an Austrian neurologist, psychiatrist, philosopher, and Holocaust survivor. He founded logotherapy, a school of psychotherapy aimed to search for a life meaning as the central human motivational force. Confronting with chaotic settings and ambiguous paths in the world, we will face frustration, stress, worry, depression, and even suicide ideation [358]. This exhausting period can be overwhelming, but resiliency and perseverance are crucial to overcoming the challenges. The positive attitude identified by Frankl, as a Holocaust survivor, is an ongoing search, which can be constellated by injuries and failures but may help in finding notes that make our experience changing life for the better. The logotherapy approach's key stroke is based on the Socratic dialogue and attitude modification. It follows the paradoxical intention and deflection by drawing attention away from the symptoms. As a pathologist and scientist, speaking of psychotherapy may be out of mind, but we, as a category, face grim and sorrows in our daily life facing with pathologies and deaths. An autopsy is the ultimate healthcare approach to the patient, trying to identify the cause of death in patients when all our knowledge and therapy modalities have been exhausted. We may approach coping with hope if we evaluate the purpose and life goals. We identify our freedom to be resilient and persist through catastrophic events. We enucleate happiness in micro-steps and develop ways to increase our courage, look for footprints of faith and belief, commit to growing, and reevaluate the hidden sides of our life and failures. Also, we discover the power of altruism, empathy, and generosity [358]. Although giving is compelling in this process of hope, it is important to realize that people in despair also need balance and clarification. In other words, we can give our wisdom or any more material gift if we establish an equation to receive from others if we allow others to enter gradually in contact with us. The anti-mask and anti-vaccine failure is associated to our response to ostracize these individuals. It is to scold some people for not wearing masks during the Capitol attack and fail to understand the anti-mask psychology [359]. As I indicated, face masks are crucial, but the common approach has contributed to a deterioration of the science behind it. Communication is key. By returning to the search for hope, it is crucial that now more than ever, during the current pandemic facing vaccine struggles and viral variants growth, we make sense of life events. We need to show to us what we want to achieve, and life purpose does not need to be written black on white, but can often be in greyAs explained in Stallone's movie, we have the choice to identify to be resilient and persist through catastrophical events freely. Here, this is an important point because it may help many teens overcome this exceedingly difficult period. Let our teenagers having the freedom to be resilient is key for our future generations. In choosing to be resilient or attempting to be persistent, we need to show that we acquire the responsibility to persist. This aspect is also crucial because it is a dynamic event, but the actor develops their responsibility, which is a very empowering feeling. There is no dichotomy between free will and responsibility but a flow, an empowering flow that may charge the individuum and increase the robustness of the soul. The enucleation of micro-steps arises from a devotion to silence the disturbing factors. A minimalist approach is important in reducing our dependence on social media and TV networks. It is important to recall the motto "Heal, Inspire, Revive" of the previous presidential campaign of the Republican Johns Hopkins neurosurgeon. The re-birth and re-empowering of conservative values are at the core of America. To move beyond our constraints, we need to understand our fallacies and take control of our decisions. Faith is not a static achievement but a dynamic process and needs to be cultivated step by step. It is not an individual decision, but a family decision and our behavior with other family components will be crucial in overcoming grief and stress. If we acknowledge that every experience is a learning opportunity, we may start identifying the fallacies as steps to improve ourselves. The commitment to growth is key in making the individuum not only stronger but more gracious person. Gracious means not only compassionate but entails the action of Lord's graces. Divine grace is a theological term not only present in Christianity but many religions. It states the Divine Influence that works in humans to revitalize and sanctify, inspire virtuous inclinations, convey strength to endure trial and resist temptation and realize the excellence of the Divine Origin. One central point of the Christian message is that "God is love" (IJn 4, 8), and a non-believer can perceive this experience through the love of his parents, relatives, and friends [360]. In Christianity, the doctrine is not built upon the experience of people giving and loving, but upon the very Divine constitution of the human being. Love is a gift that is given to us, enters us, and changes us. There is a remarkable similitude between grace and love. There is a relationship between an entity that gives and another entity that receives. It allows a verbal relationship, a dialogue, which means to speak through building a relationship. It comes from the Ancient Greek word "διάλογος." The word includes διά "through" and λόγος "speech." God's creation is for love and the reciprocity implies diffusion, i.e., our action to give the gift of our love as an expression of fraternity, communion, sociability, and solidarity (CV 34, 36, 38, 39) [360, 361]. Altruism, empathy, compassion, and generosity are powerful and develop bridges to cope with our struggles both inside of ourselves (e.g., depression and anti-mask feeling) and outside ourselves (e.g., pandemic and failure). Frankl's Socratic dialogue and attitude modification are crucial for asking ourselves about our strategy to cope with our challenges. Finally, we need to continue to appreciate what we constantly have, and we cannot reach any goal without the help of the Lord through our parents, wife, and children. By acknowledging we appreciate others and the action of our relationships and community on ourselves as small, any acknowledgment is extremely worth it. Struggle and pain are never easy to deal with, but Frankl's suggestion is to better understand living with more clarity, direction, and passion.

The Republican Party is at a decisive moment, and people with conservatory values must understand it. America and Canada need a strong Republican Party. John Danforth, a former US senator, indicates that "The Republican Party as its libertarian element present it comes across as being mean, especially in the eyes of women, minorities, and gays" in his book *The Relevance of religion*. His argumentation is not abstract but dwells in common sense that some words and actions of some republican Leaders have disaffected Independents and even some Republicans. There is a substantial opportunity in the Republican Party to correct this opinion and achieve the tremendous potential for the party and the future of the American Dream and America as a united nation. In agreement with Danforth, *The Theory of Moral Sentiments* is a critical contribution to *The Wealth of Nations*. Both documents are crucial for America, and both are not conflicting, but the practice of truth, justice, and humanity is searched. The key to reaching women, minorities, and gays effectively communicates respect, dignity, and value, because every life matters. Care is inside of the equality of the Founding Principles of most of the constitutions. The Leftists have invaded and subverted the Democratic Party, and there is no continuity with the sacred principles of the Republic that helped shaped the United States of America. For years, the Left had pursued international legitimacy rather than that of the American vote of the Middle-Class that shaped the American Dream and wanted to "de-legitimize" its opponents as "anti-Americans" because they represented the "American." Thus, the Left has abandoned the defense of the national interest. Although the Republican Party is considered under attack and de-legitimized, it is is the only party able to re-birth and continue the American Dream. Faced by insurmountable disasters and perihelic gravities in the '80s and a destabilizing political situation, Ronald Reagan, an initial Democratic Party follower, joined the Republican Party and glorified the American Dream again with respect, social progress, wordy decency, and end of the Cold War. The Democratic Party is not following the steps of the Great Fathers anymore. There is dissent in the Republican Party, but a deplorable and intrinsic crisis is present in the Democratic Party. The Democratic Party adherents do not have their own identity but are subordinate to the thought of the oligarchies and consensus generated by temporary social networks. They find themselves displaced in a world affected by challenges and no more reason for being American when they change ideas and strategies. The Republican Party needs to target and recruit more “lateral” communities. Afro-Americans, Chinese, Indians, Irish, Italians, Latinos, and First Nations among others have traditional values as the core. Black and Latino’s communities regard family and religion as a vital part of the individual’s life. Also, Muslims belong to conservatory values because their core values reside in families and hard work. The Republican Party and the Conservative Party do not belong to white citizens. Still, hard-working people of any ethnicity can find a safe place to discuss ideas and respect for traditional values. To be panglossian or bring hilarity is not the solution. Advancements may be promising, but they are ephemeral if we do not respect the thoughts of our Great Fathers. A strong America means a safer world. Americans need to reconnect to the ideals that created the most vital country that humankind ever experienced. We need to give hopes, roots and shoulders to youth shaping and consolidating the branches to discriminate between good and evil and free them from opioid and drug consumption, social media and TV networks corruption, and falsity. It is not only an arduous path but also a critical path now at the crossroad of our civilization. The hope is to reconstruct the country to freedom and pursuit of happiness that characterized the Great Fathers of the Canadian Confederation and the United States of America.

Conclusion

In this eclectic book with narrative and systematic reviews of literary and scientific knowledge, I treated the challenge of the pandemic to humanity as an essential step for a better world. In 2020, we still visualize inequalities, but the approach to it is not a "cancel culture" but a study for a better understanding of each other. We need to let people improve with the Wisdom of the humanity. In the fight against COVID-19, we emphasize the importance of testing and environmental genomics. The COVID-19 pandemic needs to be used to re-birth and re-claim our fidelity to the Fathers' spirit and bond to God. No matter how dangerous this virus is, the loss of even one life is a cry in heaven and earth. In his famous homily given on November 26th, 1981, during a liturgy for Catholic representatives of the Bundestag, which is the Lower House of the German Federal Republic, in the Church of St. Winfried [St. Boniface] in Bonn, Joseph Cardinal Ratzinger/Pope Benedict XVI commented on some crucial readings, and specifically on 1 Pet. 1:3-7 and John 14:1-6 [362]. The Church's liturgy prescribed these texts for the day. At first glance, they seemed unsuited to the subject, but following a further and closer inspection, they proved to be unexpectedly rich material for this spiritual introspection. The emeritus Pope expressed his thought in his famous speech about 40 years ago: *"The voice of Reason is never as strong as the irrational cry"* It is important to realize that *political morality consists precisely in resisting the seduction of great words.* Not the absence of any compromise, but the compromise itself is the true moral of political activity. " It is paramount to reflect on the time we live. Possible and impossible, morality and moralism, Reason and irrationality. Benedict XVI flawlessly carves the "categories" that we perceive each day conflicting heavily in the political arena. It focuses on compromise as the true moral of political activity. Yet, for many, the term compromise recalls the mess, something shady. It is not seen as a mutual commitment made by several people to act on a common interest. The moralism of the adventure, on the other hand, meets with broad consensus, as does the impossible and the unbearable. The horizon of common interest is significantly reduced, and it becomes increasingly difficult not to let oneself go to resignation or anger in the face of this truth. We will be custodians of the world and not owners if we just contemplate the Divine creation. We will need to tackle the monstruosities of capitalism and communism/socialism if we keep faith, hope, and charity in our hearts and take positive actions toward each other. The American dream will be valid for all people who will have the opportunity to raise after the failure. We must dedicate ourselves to upholding the accuracy and authority of the Scriptures, American Constitution, and the Canadian Charter of Rights and Freedoms and tireless advance to defend free speech, and encourage believers to stand firm in a dominance of obnoxious ostracism.

> "Freedom is never more than one generation away from extinction.
> We didn't pass it to our children in the bloodstream. It must be fought for, protected, and handed on for them to do the same, or one day we will spend our sunset years telling our children and our children's children what it was once like in the United States where men were free." Ronald Reagan, *A Time for Choosing*, October 27th, 1964

REFERENCES

[1] Hieronymus, ES. *De Viris Illustribus* [*On Illustrious Men*], 393.

[2] Mitchell, D. *Legacy: The Apocryphal Correspondence Between Seneca and Paul Paperback*, 2010 Aug. 3 2010.

[3] Doyle, S; Crowder, D. *Sherlock Holmes for Dummies.* Hoboken, New Jersey: John Wiley & Sons, 2010.

[4] Hochkofler, M. *Massimo Troisi*. Comico per amore 2006 Jan 1st, 2006.

[5] McDermott, JM. Joseph Ratzinger on Faith and Reason. *Angelicum.*, 2009, 86(3), 565-88. DOI, www.jstor.org/stable/44616521.

[6] Wigand, ME; Sohner, FP; Jager, M; Becker, T; Wiegand, HF. [The Dawn of Modernity: Giovanni Boccaccio's "The Decameron" and the Tradition of Genetic Understanding]. *Fortschr Neurol Psychiatr.,* 2018, 86(6), 335-41. DOI 10.1055/s-0043-119795.

[7] Cuadrada, C. [The spread of the plague: A sciento-historiographic review]. *Med Hist (Barc).*, 2015, https://www.ncbi.nlm.nih.gov/pubmed/26399143(2):4-19. DOI.

[8] Stauder, KH. [The aesculapian Decameron]. *Med Klin.*, 1958, 53(18), 802-3. DOI; https://www.ncbi.nlm.nih.gov/pubmed/13551833.

[9] Boccaccio, G. *The Decameron* [*Il Decamerone*]: Penguin Books, 1351.

[10] Sgouridou, M. The figure of the doctor and the science of medicine through Boccaccio's "Decameron". *Infez Med.,* 2014, 22(1), 62-8. DOI, https://www.ncbi.nlm.nih.gov/pubmed/24651094.

[11] Pan, X; Ojcius, DM; Gao, T; Li, Z; Pan, C; Pan, C. Lessons learned from the 2019-nCoV epidemic on prevention of future infectious diseases. *Microbes Infect.,* 2020, 22(2), 86-91. DOI 10.1016/j.micinf. 2020.02.004.

[12] Barbieri, R; Signoli, M; Cheve, D; Costedoat, C; Tzortzis, S; Aboudharam, G; Raoult, D; Drancourt, M. Yersinia pestis: the Natural History of Plague. *Clin Microbiol Rev.*, 2020, 34(1). DOI 10.1128/ CMR.00044-19.

[13] Lynteris, C. Plague Masks: The Visual Emergence of Anti-Epidemic Personal Protection Equipment. *Med Anthropol.*, 2018, 37(6), 442-57. DOI 10.1080/01459740.2017.1423072.

[14] Ahmad, T; Khan, M; Haroon, Musa TH; Nasir, S; Hui, J; Bonilla-Aldana, DK; Rodriguez-Morales, AJ. COVID-19: Zoonotic aspects. *Travel Med Infect Dis.,* 2020, 10.1016/j.tmaid.2020.101607:101607. DOI 10.1016/j.tmaid.2020.101607.

[15] Butler, T. Plague history: Yersin's discovery of the causative bacterium in 1894 enabled, in the subsequent century, scientific progress in understanding the disease and the development of treatments and vaccines. *Clin Microbiol Infect.,* 2014, 20(3), 202-9. DOI 10.1111/1469-0691.12540.

[16] CDC. *8 Zoonotic Diseases Shared Between Animals and People of Most Concern in the U.S. 2019.* DOI; https://www.cdc.gov/ media/releases/2019/s0506-zoonotic-diseases-shared.html.

[17] Ahmad, T; Hui, J. One Health approach and Coronavirus Disease 2019. *Hum Vaccin Immunother.*, 2020, 10.1080/ 21645515.2020. 1732168:1-2. DOI 10.1080/21645515.2020.1732168.

[18] Bassareo, PP; Melis, MR; Marras, S; Calcaterra, G. Learning from the past in the COVID-19 era: rediscovery of quarantine, previous pandemics, origin of hospitals and national healthcare systems, and ethics in medicine. *Postgrad Med J.,* 2020, 96(1140), 633-8. DOI 10.1136/postgradmedj-2020-138370.

[19] Kilwein, JH. Some historical comments on quarantine: Part One. *J Clin Pharm Ther.,* 1995, 20(4), 185-7. DOI 10.1111/j.1365-2710.1995.tb00647.x.

[20] Sergi, C. *Pathology of Childhood and Adolescence*. 1st ed: Springer, 2020 October 29, 2020.

[21] Scott, S; Duncan, C. *Biology of plagues: evidence from historical populations*. Philadelphia, PA, USA: University of Pennsylvania Press; 2001.

[22] Griffin, M; Sohrabi, C; Alsafi, Z; Nicola, M; Kerwan, A; Mathew, G; Agha, R. Preparing for COVID-19 exit strategies. *Ann Med Surg* (Lond)., 2021, 61, 88-92. DOI 10.1016/j.amsu.2020.12.012.

[23] Iacobucci, G. Covid-19: UK lockdown is "crucial" to saving lives; say doctors and scientists. *BMJ*., 2020, 368, m1204. DOI 10.1136/ bmj.m1204.

[24] Ji, T; Chen, HL; Xu, J; Wu, LN; Li, JJ; Chen, K; Qin, G. Lockdown contained the spread of 2019 novel coronavirus disease in Huangshi city, China: Early epidemiological findings. *Clin Infect Dis*., 2020, 10.1093/cid/ciaa390. DOI 10.1093/cid/ciaa390.

[25] Angeletti, LR; Gazzaniga, V. [The plague of Syracuse (396 B.C.E.) in Diodorus Siculus (XIV, 70)]. *Ann Ig*., 2002, 14(1 Suppl 1), 7-13. DOI; https://www.ncbi.nlm.nih.gov/pubmed/12162139.

[26] Harper, K. Chapter 4: *The Old Age of the World. The Fate of Rome: Climate, Disease, and the End of an Empire*.: Princeton University Press., 2017.

[27] Harper, K. Solving the Mystery of an Ancient Roman Plague. *The Atlantic.,* November 1, 2017.

[28] Cicero, MT. *De oratore*. Leipzig (Germany): B.G. Teubner, 1862, 471 p.

[29] Cicero, MT. *On oratory and orators*. New York, NY, USA: Harper & Brothers., 1860.

[30] LePan, N. Visualizing the History of Pandemics. *Visual Capitalist* [Internet]., 2020, February 7, 2021, https://www.visualcapitalist.com/ history-of-pandemics-deadliest/. Available from: https://www.visual capitalist.com/history-of-pandemics-deadliest/.

[31] Serra, N; Di Carlo, P; Rea, T; Sergi, CM. Diffusion modeling of COVID-19 under lockdown. *Physics of Fluids* [Internet]., 2021, 33, [041903 p.]. Available from: https://doi.org/10.1063/5.0044061.

[32] Aronna, MS; Guglielmi, R; Moschen, LM. A model for COVID-19 with isolation, quarantine and testing as control measures. *Epidemics*., 2021, 34, 100437. DOI 10.1016/j.epidem.2021.100437.

[33] Viceconte, G; Petrosillo, N. COVID-19 R0: Magic number or conundrum? *Infect Dis Rep*., 2020, 12(1), 8516. DOI 10.4081/idr.2020.8516.

[34] Chen, TM; Rui, J; Wang, QP; Zhao, ZY; Cui, JA; Yin, L. A mathematical model for simulating the phase-based transmissibility of a novel coronavirus. *Infect Dis Poverty.,* 2020, 9(1), 24. DOI 10.1186/s40249-020-00640-3.

[35] Magner, LN. *A History of Medicine.* New York, NY, U.S.A.: Marcel Dekker, Inc., 1992.

[36] Greenstone, G. The history of bloodletting. *BCMJ*., 2010, 52(1), 12-4. DOI.

[37] Labadie, T; Batejat, C; Leclercq, I; Manuguerra, JC. Historical Discoveries on Viruses in the Environment and Their Impact on Public Health. *Intervirology*., 2020, 63(1-6), 17-32. DOI 10.1159/000511575.

[38] Sergi, C. Diversity, Cultural Competence, and Multiculturalism: A Stronghold for the Future of Biotechnology. *Ann Clin Lab Sci*., 2018, 48(4), 549-52. DOI; https://www.ncbi.nlm.nih.gov/pubmed/30143502.

[39] Chen, JD; Xu, H. Historical development of Chinese dietary patterns and nutrition from the ancient to the modern society. *World Rev Nutr Diet*., 1996, 79, 133-53. DOI 10.1159/000425370.

[40] Gasbarrini, G; Bonvicini, F; Gramenzi, A. Probiotics History. *J Clin Gastroenterol.*, 2016, 50 Suppl 2, *Proceedings from the 8th Probiotics, Prebiotics & New Foods for Microbiota and Human Health* meeting held in Rome, Italy on September 13-15, 2015, S116-S9. DOI 10.1097/MCG.0000000000000697.

[41] Solos, I; Liang, Y. A historical evaluation of Chinese tongue diagnosis in the treatment of septicemic plague in the pre-antibiotic era, and as a new direction for revolutionary clinical research applications. *J Integr Med*., 2018, 16(3), 141-6. DOI 10.1016/j.joim.2018.04.001.

[42] Teng, L; Zu, Q; Li, G; Yu, T; Job, KM; Yang, X; Di, L; Sherwin, CM; Enioutina, EY. Herbal medicines: challenges in the modern world. Part 3. China and Japan. *Expert Rev Clin Pharmacol.*, 2016, 9(9), 1225-33. DOI 10.1080/17512433.2016.1195263.

[43] Fu, L. Surgical history of ancient China: Part 2. *ANZ J Surg.*, 2010, 80(3), 133-8. DOI 10.1111/j.1445-2197.2010.05212.x.

[44] Fu, L. Surgical history of ancient China: part 1. *ANZ J Surg.*, 2009, 79(12), 879-85. DOI 10.1111/j.1445-2197.2009.05138.x.

[45] Murphy, FA. The threat posed by the global emergence of livestock, food-borne, and zoonotic pathogens. *Ann N Y Acad Sci.*, 1999, 894, 20-7. DOI 10.1111/j.1749-6632.1999.tb08039.x.

[46] Cloeckaert, A. Introduction: emerging antimicrobial resistance mechanisms in the zoonotic foodborne pathogens Salmonella and Campylobacter. *Microbes Infect.,* 2006, 8(7), 1889-90. DOI 10.1016/j.micinf.2005.12.024.

[47] Humphrey, T; O'Brien, S; Madsen, M. Campylobacters as zoonotic pathogens: a food production perspective. *Int J Food Microbiol.*, 2007, 117(3), 237-57. DOI 10.1016/j.ijfoodmicro.2007.01.006.

[48] Scotch, M; Brownstein, JS; Vegso, S; Galusha, D; Rabinowitz, P. Human vs. animal outbreaks of the 2009 swine-origin H1N1 influenza A epidemic. *Ecohealth.*, 2011, 8(3), 376-80. DOI 10.1007/s10393-011-0706-x.

[49] Wang, WH; Urbina, AN; Chang, MR; Assavalapsakul, W; Lu, PL; Chen, YH; Wang, SF. Dengue hemorrhagic fever - A systemic literature review of current perspectives on pathogenesis, prevention and control. *J Microbiol Immunol Infect.*, 2020, 53(6), 963-78. DOI 10.1016/j.jmii.2020.03.007.

[50] Derraik, JGB; Anderson, WA; Connelly, EA; Anderson, YC. Rapid Review of SARS-CoV-1 and SARS-CoV-2 Viability, Susceptibility to Treatment, and the Disinfection and Reuse of PPE, Particularly Filtering Facepiece Respirators. *Int J Environ Res Public Health.*, 2020, 17(17). DOI 10.3390/ijerph17176117.

[51] Burnett, ML; Sergi, CM. Face Masks are Beneficial Regardless of the Level of Infection in the Fight Against COVID-19. *Disaster Med*

Public Health Prep., 2020, 10.1017/dmp.2020.320:1-13. DOI 10.1017/dmp.2020.320.

[52] Ciotti, M; Angeletti, S; Minieri, M; Giovannetti, M; Benvenuto, D; Pascarella, S; Sagnelli, C; Bianchi, M; Bernardini, S; Ciccozzi, M. COVID-19 Outbreak: An Overview. *Chemotherapy.*, 2020, 10.1159/000507423:1-9. DOI 10.1159/000507423.

[53] Khan, A; Sergi, C. SAMHD1 as the Potential Link Between SARS-CoV-2 Infection and Neurological Complications. *Front Neurol.*, 2020, 11, 562913. DOI 10.3389/fneur.2020.562913.

[54] Rodriguez-Morales, AJ; Gallego, V; Escalera-Antezana, JP; Mendez, CA; Zambrano, LI; Franco-Paredes, C; Suarez, JA; Rodriguez-Enciso, HD; Balbin-Ramon, GJ; Savio-Larriera, E; Risquez, A; Cimerman, S. COVID-19 in Latin America: The implications of the first confirmed case in Brazil. *Travel Med Infect Dis.*, 2020, 10.1016/j.tmaid.2020.101613:101613. DOI 10.1016/ j.tmaid.2020.101613.

[55] Sergi, CM; Chiu, B. Targeting NLRP3 inflammasome in an animal model for Coronavirus Disease 2019 (COVID-19) caused by the Severe Acute Respiratory Syndrome Coronavirus 2 (SARS-CoV-2). *J Med Virol.*, 2020, 10.1002/jmv.26461. DOI 10.1002/jmv.26461.

[56] Cascella, M; Rajnik, M; Cuomo, A; Dulebohn, SC; Di Napoli, R. *Features, Evaluation and Treatment Coronavirus* (COVID-19). StatPearls, https://www.ncbi.nlm.nih.gov/pubmed/32150360. Treasure Island (FL)2020.

[57] Rothan, HA; Byrareddy, SN. The epidemiology and pathogenesis of coronavirus disease (COVID-19) outbreak. *J Autoimmun.*, 2020, 10.1016/j.jaut.2020.102433:102433. DOI 10.1016/j.jaut.2020. 102433.

[58] He, F; Deng, Y; Li, W. Coronavirus disease 2019: What we know? *J Med Virol.*, 2020, 10.1002/jmv.25766. DOI 10.1002/jmv.25766.

[59] Bernard Stoecklin, S; Rolland, P; Silue, Y; Mailles, A; Campese, C; Simondon, A; Mechain, M; Meurice, L; Nguyen, M; Bassi, C; Yamani, E; Behillil, S; Ismael, S; Nguyen, D; Malvy, D; Lescure, FX; Georges, S; Lazarus, C; Tabai, A; Stempfelet, M; Enouf, V; Coignard, B; Levy-Bruhl, D; Investigation, T. First cases of coronavirus disease

2019 (COVID-19) in France: surveillance, investigations and control measures, January 2020. *Euro Surveill.*, 2020, 25(6). DOI 10.2807/1560-7917.ES.2020.25.6.2000094.

[60] Spiteri, G; Fielding, J; Diercke, M; Campese, C; Enouf, V; Gaymard, A; Bella, A; Sognamiglio, P; Sierra Moros, MJ; Riutort, AN; Demina, YV; Mahieu, R; Broas, M; Bengner, M; Buda, S; Schilling, J; Filleul, L; Lepoutre, A; Saura, C; Mailles, A; Levy-Bruhl, D; Coignard, B; Bernard-Stoecklin, S; Behillil, S; van der Werf, S; Valette, M; Lina, B; Riccardo, F; Nicastri, E; Casas, I; Larrauri, A; Salom Castell, M; Pozo, F; Maksyutov, RA; Martin, C; Van Ranst, M; Bossuyt, N; Siira, L; Sane, J; Tegmark-Wisell, K; Palmerus, M; Broberg, EK; Beaute, J; Jorgensen, P; Bundle, N; Pereyaslov, D; Adlhoch, C; Pukkila, J; Pebody, R; Olsen, S; Ciancio, BC. First cases of coronavirus disease 2019 (COVID-19) in the WHO European Region, 24 January to 21 February 2020. *Euro Surveill.*, 2020, 25(9). DOI 10.2807/1560-7917.ES.2020.25.9.2000178.

[61] Lai, CC; Liu, YH; Wang, CY; Wang, YH; Hsueh, SC; Yen, MY; Ko, WC; Hsueh, PR. Asymptomatic carrier state, acute respiratory disease, and pneumonia due to severe acute respiratory syndrome coronavirus 2 (SARS-CoV-2): Facts and myths. *J Microbiol Immunol Infect.*, 2020, 10.1016/j.jmii.2020.02.012. DOI 10.1016/j.jmii.2020.02.012.

[62] Tian, S; Xiong, Y; Liu, H; Niu, L; Guo, J; Liao, M; Xiao, SY. Pathological study of the 2019 novel coronavirus disease (COVID-19) through postmortem core biopsies. *Mod Pathol.*, 2020, 33(6), 1007-14. DOI 10.1038/s41379-020-0536-x.

[63] Rubin, GD; Haramati, LB; Kanne, JP; Schluger, NW; Yim, JJ; Anderson, DJ; Altes, T; Desai, SR; Goo, JM; Inoue, Y; Luo, F; Prokop, M; Richeldi, L; Tomiyama, N; Leung, AN; Ryerson, CJ; Sverzellati, N; Raoof, S; Volpi, A; Martin, IBK; Kong, C; Bush, A; Goldin, J; Humbert, M; Kauczor, HU; Mazzone, PJ; Remy-Jardin, M; Schaefer-Prokop, CM; Wells, AU. The Role of Chest Imaging in Patient Management during the COVID-19 Pandemic: A Multinational Consensus Statement from the Fleischner Society. *Radiology.*,

2020, 10.1148/radiol.2020201365:201365. DOI 10.1148/radiol. 2020201365.

[64] Hanley, B; Lucas, SB; Youd, E; Swift, B; Osborn, M. Autopsy in suspected COVID-19 cases. *J Clin Pathol.*, 2020, 10.1136/jclinpath-2020-206522. DOI 10.1136/jclinpath-2020-206522.

[65] Lin, X; Gong, Z; Xiao, Z; Xiong, J; Fan, B; Liu, J. Novel Coronavirus Pneumonia Outbreak in 2019: Computed Tomographic Findings in Two Cases. *Korean J Radiol.,* 2020, 21(3), 365-8. DOI 10.3348/kjr.2020.0078.

[66] Ackermann, M; Verleden, SE; Kuehnel, M; Haverich, A; Welte, T; Laenger, F; Vanstapel, A; Werlein, C; Stark, H; Tzankov, A; Li, WW; Li, VW; Mentzer, SJ; Jonigk, D. Pulmonary Vascular Endothelialitis, Thrombosis, and Angiogenesis in Covid-19. *N Engl J Med.*, 2020, 383(2), 120-8. DOI 10.1056/NEJMoa2015432.

[67] Bansal, M. Cardiovascular disease and COVID-19. *Diabetes Metab Syndr.*, 2020, 14(3), 247-50. DOI 10.1016/j.dsx.2020.03.013.

[68] Burnett, ML; Sergi, CM. Face Masks Are Beneficial Regardless of the Level of Infection in the Fight Against COVID-19. *Disaster Med Public Health Prep.*, 2020, 14(5), e47-e50. DOI 10.1017/ dmp.2020.320.

[69] Sergi, CM; Leung, AKC. The facemask in public and healthcare workers: a need, not a belief. *Public Health.*, 2020, 183, 67-8. DOI 10.1016/j.puhe.2020.05.009.

[70] Cheng, VCC; Wong, SC; Chen, JHK; Yip, CCY; Chuang, VWM; Tsang, OTY; Sridhar, S; Chan, JFW; Ho, PL; Yuen, KY. Escalating infection control response to the rapidly evolving epidemiology of the coronavirus disease 2019 (COVID-19) due to SARS-CoV-2 in Hong Kong. *Infect Control Hosp Epidemiol.*, 2020, 10.1017/ice.2020.58:1-6. DOI 10.1017/ice.2020.58.

[71] Ferioli, M; Cisternino, C; Leo, V; Pisani, L; Palange, P; Nava, S. Protecting healthcare workers from SARS-CoV-2 infection: practical indications. *Eur Respir Rev.*, 2020, 29(155). DOI 10.1183/16000617.0068-2020.

[72] Wong, SC; Kwong, RT; Wu, TC; Chan, JWM; Chu, MY; Lee, SY; Wong, HY; Lung, DC. Risk of nosocomial transmission of coronavirus disease 2019: an experience in a general ward setting in Hong Kong. *J Hosp Infect.*, 2020, 10.1016/j.jhin.2020.03.036. DOI 10.1016/j.jhin.2020.03.036.

[73] Kampf, G; Todt, D; Pfaender, S; Steinmann, E. Persistence of coronaviruses on inanimate surfaces and their inactivation with biocidal agents. *J Hosp Infect.*, 2020, 104(3), 246-51. DOI 10.1016/j.jhin.2020.01.022.

[74] To, KK; Tsang, OT; Leung, WS; Tam, AR; Wu, TC; Lung, DC; Yip, CC; Cai, JP; Chan, JM; Chik, TS; Lau, DP; Choi, CY; Chen, LL; Chan, WM; Chan, KH; Ip, JD; Ng, AC; Poon, RW; Luo, CT; Cheng, VC; Chan, JF; Hung, IF; Chen, Z; Chen, H; Yuen, KY. Temporal profiles of viral load in posterior oropharyngeal saliva samples and serum antibody responses during infection by SARS-CoV-2: an observational cohort study. *Lancet Infect Dis.*, 2020, 10.1016/S1473-3099(20)30196-1. DOI 10.1016/S1473-3099(20)30196-1.

[75] Zhai, P; Ding, Y; Wu, X; Long, J; Zhong, Y; Li, Y. The epidemiology; diagnosis and treatment of COVID-19. *Int J Antimicrob Agents.*, 2020, 10.1016/ j.ijantimicag.2020.105955:105955. DOI 10.1016/ j.ijantimicag.2020.105955.

[76] CDC. Evidence used to update the list of underlying medical conditions that increase a person's risk of severe illness from COVID-19. *COVID-19* [Internet]., 2020 Mar 11, 2021, https://www.cdc.gov/coronavirus/2019-ncov/need-extra-precautions/evidence-table.html#print. Available from: https://www.cdc.gov/ coronavirus/2019-ncov/need-extra-precautions/evidence-table.html#print.

[77] De Toma, I; Dierssen, M. Network analysis of Down syndrome and SARS-CoV-2 identifies risk and protective factors for COVID-19. *Sci Rep.*, 2021, 11(1), 1930. DOI 10.1038/s41598-021-81451-w.

[78] Coperchini, F; Chiovato, L; Croce, L; Magri, F; Rotondi, M. The cytokine storm in COVID-19: An overview of the involvement of the chemokine/chemokine-receptor system. *Cytokine Growth Factor Rev.*, 2020, 53, 25-32. DOI 10.1016/j.cytogfr.2020.05.003.

[79] Glass, WG; Subbarao, K; Murphy, B; Murphy, PM. Mechanisms of host defense following severe acute respiratory syndrome-coronavirus (SARS-CoV) pulmonary infection of mice. *J Immunol.*, 2004, 173(6):4030-9. DOI 10.4049/jimmunol.173.6.4030.

[80] Xiong, Y; Liu, Y; Cao, L; Wang, D; Guo, M; Jiang, A; Guo, D; Hu, W; Yang, J; Tang, Z; Wu, H; Lin, Y; Zhang, M; Zhang, Q; Shi, M; Liu, Y; Zhou, Y; Lan, K; Chen, Y. Transcriptomic characteristics of bronchoalveolar lavage fluid and peripheral blood mononuclear cells in COVID-19 patients. *Emerg Microbes Infect.*, 2020, 9(1), 761-70. DOI 10.1080/22221751.2020.1747363.

[81] Alipour, M; Zaidi, D; Valcheva, R; Jovel, J; Martinez, I; Sergi, C; Walter, J; Mason, AL; Wong, GK; Dieleman, LA; Carroll, MW; Huynh, HQ; Wine, E. Mucosal Barrier Depletion and Loss of Bacterial Diversity are Primary Abnormalities in Paediatric Ulcerative Colitis. *J Crohns Colitis.*, 2016, 10(4), 462-71. DOI 10.1093/ecco-jcc/jjv223.

[82] Alipour, M; Lou, Y; Zimmerman, D; Bording-Jorgensen, MW; Sergi, C; Liu, JJ; Wine, E. A balanced IL-1beta activity is required for host response to Citrobacter rodentium infection. *PLoS One.*, 2013, 8(12), e80656. DOI 10.1371/journal.pone.0080656.

[83] NIH. Coronavirus Disease 2019 (COVID-19) *Treatment Guidelines*, 2021 Mar 11, 2021, https://www.covid19treatmentguidelines.nih.gov/. Available from: https://www.covid19treatmentguidelines.nih.gov/.

[84] Al-Horani, RA; Kar, S. Potential Anti-SARS-CoV-2 Therapeutics That Target the Post-Entry Stages of the Viral Life Cycle: A Comprehensive Review. *Viruses.*, 2020, 12(10). DOI 10.3390/v12101092.

[85] Zhang, C; Huang, S; Zheng, F; Dai, Y. Controversial treatments: an updated understanding of the Coronavirus Disease 2019. *J Med Virol.*, 2020, 10.1002/jmv.25788. DOI 10.1002/jmv.25788.

[86] Cao, YC; Deng, QX; Dai, SX. Remdesivir for severe acute respiratory syndrome coronavirus 2 causing COVID-19: An evaluation of the evidence. *Travel Med Infect Dis.*, 2020, 10.1016/j.tmaid.2020.101647:101647. DOI 10.1016/j.tmaid.2020.101647.

[87] Albariqi, AH; Chang, RYK; Tai, W; Ke, WR; Chow, MYT; Tang, P; Kwok, PCL; Chan, HK. Inhalable Hydroxychloroquine Powders for Potential Treatment of COVID-19. *J Aerosol Med Pulm Drug Deliv.*, 2021, 34(1), 20-31. DOI 10.1089/jamp.2020.1648.

[88] Barlow, A; Landolf, KM; Barlow, B; Yeung, SYA; Heavner, JJ; Claassen, CW; Heavner, MS. Review of Emerging Pharmacotherapy for the Treatment of Coronavirus Disease 2019. *Pharmacotherapy.*, 2020, 10.1002/phar.2398. DOI 10.1002/phar.2398.

[89] Cusinato, J; Cau, Y; Calvani, AM; Mori, M. Repurposing drugs for the management of COVID-19. *Expert Opin Ther Pat.*, 2020, 10.1080/13543776.2021.1861248:1-13. DOI 10.1080/ 13543776. 2021.1861248.

[90] Thakur, S; Mayank, Sarkar B; Ansari, AJ; Khandelwal, A; Arya, A; Poduri, R; Joshi, G. Exploring the magic bullets to identify Achilles' heel in SARS-CoV-2: Delving deeper into the sea of possible therapeutic options in Covid-19 disease: An update. *Food Chem Toxicol.*, 2021, 147, 111887. DOI 10.1016/j.fct.2020.111887.

[91] Meng, L; Qiu, H; Wan, L; Ai, Y; Xue, Z; Guo, Q; Deshpande, R; Zhang, L; Meng, J; Tong, C; Liu, H; Xiong, L. Intubation and Ventilation amid the COVID-19 Outbreak: Wuhan's Experience. *Anesthesiology.*, 2020, 10.1097/ALN.0000000000003296. DOI 10.1097/ALN.0000000000003296,

[92] Lucchesi, A; Silimbani, P; Musuraca, G; Cerchione, C; Martinelli, G; Di Carlo, P; Napolitano, M. Clinical and biological data on the use of hydroxychloroquine against SARS-CoV-2 could support the role of the NLRP3 inflammasome in the pathogenesis of respiratory disease. *J Med Virol.,* 2020, 10.1002/jmv.26217. DOI 10.1002/jmv.26217.

[93] Freeman, TL; Swartz, TH. Targeting the NLRP3 Inflammasome in Severe COVID-19. *Front Immunol.*, 2020, 11, 1518. DOI 10.3389/fimmu.2020.01518.

[94] Colantuoni, A; Martini, R; Caprari, P; Ballestri, M; Capecchi, PL; Gnasso, A; Lo Presti, R; Marcoccia, A; Rossi, M; Caimi, G. COVID-19 Sepsis and Microcirculation Dysfunction. *Front Physiol.*, 2020, 11, 747. DOI 10.3389/fphys.2020.00747.

[95] He, L; Ding, Y; Zhang, Q; Che, X; He, Y; Shen, H, Wang, H; Li, Z; Zhao, L; Geng, J; Deng, Y; Yang, L; Li, J; Cai, J; Qiu, L; Wen, K; Xu, X; Jiang, S. Expression of elevated levels of pro-inflammatory cytokines in SARS-CoV-infected ACE2+ cells in SARS patients: relation to the acute lung injury and pathogenesis of SARS. *J Pathol.*, 2006, 210(3), 288-97. DOI 10.1002/path.2067.

[96] Chiu, B; Jantuan, E; Shen, F; Chiu, B; Sergi, C. Autophagy-Inflammasome Interplay in Heart Failure: A Systematic Review on Basics, Pathways, and Therapeutic Perspectives. *Ann Clin Lab Sci.*, 2017, 47(3), 243-52. DOI; https://www.ncbi.nlm.nih.gov/pubmed/28667023.

[97] Ahlawat, S; Asha, Sharma KK. Immunological co-ordination between gut and lungs in SARS-CoV-2 infection. *Virus Res.*, 2020, 286, 198103. DOI 10.1016/j.virusres.2020.198103.

[98] Cha, MH; Regueiro, M; Sandhu, DS. Gastrointestinal and hepatic manifestations of COVID-19: A comprehensive review. *World J Gastroenterol.*, 2020, 26(19), 2323-32. DOI 10.3748/wjg.v26.i19.2323.

[99] Geddes, K; Rubino, SJ; Magalhaes, JG; Streutker, C; Le Bourhis, L; Cho, JH; Robertson, SJ; Kim, CJ; Kaul, R; Philpott, DJ; Girardin, SE. Identification of an innate T helper type 17 response to intestinal bacterial pathogens. *Nat Med.*, 2011, 17(7), 837-44. DOI 10.1038/nm.2391.

[100] Wu, F; Zhao, S; Yu, B; Chen, YM; Wang, W; Song, ZG; Hu, Y; Tao, ZW; Tian, JH; Pei, YY; Yuan, ML; Zhang, YL; Dai, FH; Liu, Y; Wang, QM; Zheng, JJ; Xu, L; Holmes, EC; Zhang, YZ. A new coronavirus associated with human respiratory disease in China. *Nature.*, 2020, 579(7798), 265-9. DOI 10.1038/s41586-020-2008-3.

[101] Wang, MY; Zhao, R; Gao, LJ; Gao, XF; Wang, DP; Cao, JM. SARS-CoV-2: Structure, Biology, and Structure-Based Therapeutics Development. *Front Cell Infect Microbiol.,* 2020, 10, 587269. DOI 10.3389/fcimb.2020.587269

[102] Lu, R; Zhao, X; Li, J; Niu, P; Yang, B; Wu, H; Wang, W; Song, H; Huang, B; Zhu, N; Bi, Y; Ma, X; Zhan, F; Wang, L; Hu, T; Zhou, H;

Hu, Z; Zhou, W; Zhao, L; Chen, J; Meng, Y; Wang, J; Lin, Y; Yuan, J; Xie, Z; Ma, J; Liu, WJ; Wang, D; Xu, W; Holmes, EC; Gao, GF, Wu, G; Chen, W; Shi, W; Tan, W. Genomic characterisation and epidemiology of 2019 novel coronavirus: implications for virus origins and receptor binding. *Lancet.*, 2020, 395(10224), 565-74. DOI 10.1016/S0140-6736(20)30251-8

[103] O'Leary, VB; Dolly, OJ; Hoschl, C; Cerna, M; Ovsepian, SV. Unpacking Pandora From Its Box: Deciphering the Molecular Basis of the SARS-CoV-2 Coronavirus. *Int J Mol Sci.*, 2020, 22(1). DOI 10.3390/ijms22010386.

[104] Zhou, P; Yang, XL; Wang, XG; Hu, B; Zhang, L; Zhang, W; Si, HR; Zhu, Y; Li, B; Huang, CL; Chen, HD; Chen, J; Luo, Y; Guo, H; Jiang, RD; Liu, MQ; Chen, Y; Shen, XR; Wang, X; Zheng, XS; Zhao, K; Chen, QJ; Deng, F; Liu, LL; Yan, B; Zhan, FX; Wang, YY; Xiao, GF; Shi, ZL. A pneumonia outbreak associated with a new coronavirus of probable bat origin. *Nature.*, 2020, 579(7798), 270-3. DOI 10.1038/s41586-020-2012-7.

[105] Zhang, C; Zheng, W; Huang, X; Bell, EW; Zhou, X; Zhang, Y. Protein Structure and Sequence Reanalysis of 2019-nCoV Genome Refutes Snakes as Its Intermediate Host and the Unique Similarity between Its Spike Protein Insertions and HIV-1. *J Proteome Res.*, 2020, 19(4), 1351-60. DOI 10.1021/acs.jproteome.0c00129.

[106] Ralph, R; Lew, J; Zeng, T; Francis, M; Xue, B; Roux, M; Toloue, Ostadgavahi, A; Rubino, S; Dawe, NJ; Al-Ahdal, MN; Kelvin, DJ; Richardson, CD; Kindrachuk, J; Falzarano, D; Kelvin, AA. 2019-nCoV (Wuhan virus), a novel Coronavirus: human-to-human transmission, travel-related cases, and vaccine readiness. *J Infect Dev Ctries.*, 2020, 14(1), 3-17. DOI 10.3855/jidc.12425.

[107] Borges do Nascimento, IJ; Cacic, N; Abdulazeem, HM; von Groote, TC; Jayarajah, U; Weerasekara, I; Esfahani, MA; Civile, VT; Marusic, A; Jeroncic, A; Carvas Junior, N; Pericic, TP; Zakarija-Grkovic, I; Meirelles Guimaraes, SM; Luigi Bragazzi, N; Bjorklund, M; Sofi-Mahmudi, A; Altujjar, M; Tian, M; Arcani, DMC; O'Mathuna, DP; Marcolino, MS. Novel Coronavirus Infection

(COVID-19) in Humans: A Scoping Review and Meta-Analysis. *J Clin Med.*, 2020, 9(4). DOI 10.3390/jcm9040941.

[108] Burnett, M; Abuetabh, Y; Wronski, A; Shen, F; Persad, S; Leng, R; Eisenstat, D; Sergi, C. Graphene Oxide Nanoparticles Induce Apoptosis in wild-type and CRISPR/Cas9-IGF/IGFBP3 knocked-out Osteosarcoma Cells. *J Cancer.*, 2020, 11(17), 5007-23. DOI 10.7150/jca.46464.

[109] Yuce, M; Filiztekin, E; Ozkaya, KG. COVID-19 diagnosis -A review of current methods. *Biosens Bioelectron.,* 2021, 172, 112752. DOI 10.1016/j.bios.2020.112752.

[110] Li, Z; Yi, Y; Luo, X; Xiong, N; Liu, Y; Li, S; Sun, R; Wang, Y; Hu, B; Chen, W; Zhang, Y; Wang, J; Huang, B; Lin, Y; Yang, J; Cai, W; Wang, X; Cheng, J; Chen, Z; Sun, K; Pan, W; Zhan, Z; Chen, L; Ye, F. Development and Clinical Application of A Rapid IgM-IgG Combined Antibody Test for SARS-CoV-2 Infection Diagnosis. *J Med Virol.*, 2020, 10.1002/jmv.25727. DOI 10.1002/jmv.25727.

[111] Verkerke, H; Horwath, M; Saeedi, B; Boyer, D; Allen, JW; Owens, J; Arthur, CM; Nakahara, H; Rha, J; Patel, K; Wu, SC; Paul, A; Yasin, N; Wang, J; Shin, S; Brown, D; Normile, K; Cole, L; Meyers, M; Lin, H; Woods, E; Isaac, J; Broder, K; Wade, J; Kauffman, RC; Patel, R; Josephson, CD; Reynolds, S; Sherman, M; Wrammert, J; Alter, D; Guarner, J; Roback, JD; Neish, A; Stowell, SR. Comparison of Antibody Class Specific SARS-CoV-2 Serology for the Diagnosis of Acute COVID-19. *J Clin Microbiol.*, 2021, 10.1128/JCM.02026-20. DOI 10.1128/JCM.02026-20.

[112] Verma, N; Patel, D; Pandya, A. Emerging diagnostic tools for detection of COVID-19 and perspective. *Biomed Microdevices.*, 2020, 22(4), 83. DOI 10.1007/s10544-020-00534-z.

[113] Moulahoum, H; Ghorbanizamani, F; Zihnioglu, F; Turhan, K; Timur, S. How should diagnostic kits development adapt quickly in COVID 19-like pandemic models? Pros and cons of sensory platforms used in COVID-19 sensing. *Talanta.*, 2021, 222, 121534. DOI 10.1016/j.talanta.2020.121534.

[114] Kitsios, GD; Bain, W; Al-Yousif, N; Duttagupta, R; Ahmed, AA; McVerry, BJ; Morris, A. Plasma microbial cell-free DNA load is associated with mortality in patients with COVID-19. *Respir Res.*, 2021, 22(1), 24. DOI 10.1186/s12931-021-01623-0.

[115] Arunachalam, PS; Wimmers, F; Mok, CKP; Perera, R; Scott, M; Hagan, T; Sigal, N; Feng, Y; Bristow, L; Tak-Yin Tsang, O; Wagh, D; Coller, J; Pellegrini, KL; Kazmin, D; Alaaeddine, G; Leung, WS; Chan, JMC; Chik, TSH; Choi, CYC; Huerta, C; Paine, McCullough, M; Lv, H; Anderson, E; Edupuganti, S; Upadhyay, AA; Bosinger, SE; Maecker, HT; Khatri, P; Rouphael, N; Peiris, M; Pulendran, B. Systems biological assessment of immunity to mild versus severe COVID-19 infection in humans. *Science.*, 2020, 369(6508), 1210-20. DOI 10.1126/science.abc6261.

[116] Gu, W; Miller, S; Chiu, CY. Clinical Metagenomic Next-Generation Sequencing for Pathogen Detection. *Annu Rev Pathol.*, 2019, 14, 319-38. DOI 10.1146/annurev-pathmechdis-012418-012751.

[117] Carbo, EC; Sidorov, IA; Zevenhoven-Dobbe, JC; Snijder, EJ; Claas, EC; Laros, JFJ; Kroes, ACM; de Vries, JJC. Coronavirus discovery by metagenomic sequencing: a tool for pandemic preparedness. *J Clin Virol.*, 2020, 131, 104594. DOI 10.1016/j.jcv.2020.104594.

[118] Lam, TT; Shum, MH; Zhu, HC; Tong, YG; Ni, XB; Liao, YS; Wei, W; Cheung, WY; Li, WJ; Li, LF; Leung, GM; Holmes, EC; Hu, YL; Guan, Y. Identifying SARS-CoV-2 related coronaviruses in Malayan pangolins. *Nature.*, 2020, 10.1038/s41586-020-2169-0. DOI 10.1038/s41586-020-2169-0.

[119] Sawyer, A; Free, T; Martin, J. Metagenomics: preventing future pandemics. *Biotechniques.*, 2021, 70(1), 1-4. DOI 10.2144/btn-2020-0166.

[120] Mohseni, H; Amini, S; Abiri, B; Kalantar, M; Kaydani, M; Barati, B; Pirabbasi, E; Bahrami, F. Are history of dietary intake and food habits of patients with clinical symptoms of COVID 19 different from healthy controls? A case-control study. *Clin Nutr ESPEN.*, 2021, 42, 280-5. DOI 10.1016/j.clnesp.2021.01.021.

[121] Fitzgerald, M; Thornton, L; O'Gorman, J; O'Connor, L; Garvey, P; Boland, M; Part, AM; Rogalska, J; Coughlan, H; MacDiarmadam J; Heslin, J; Canny, M; Finnegan, P; Moran, J; O'Flanagan, D; Hepatitis, AOCT. Outbreak of hepatitis A infection associated with the consumption of frozen berries, Ireland, 2013--linked to an international outbreak. *Euro Surveill.,* 2014, 19(43). DOI 10.2807/1560-7917.es2014.19.43.20942.

[122] Kim, DH; Chung, WC; Chun, SH; Han, JH; Song, MJ; Lee, KW. Enhancing the natural killer cell activity and anti-influenza effect of heat-treated Lactobacillus plantarum nF1-fortified yogurt in mice. *J Dairy Sci*., 2018, 101(12), 10675-84. DOI 10.3168/jds.2018-15137.

[123] Kaila, M; Isolauri, E; Soppi, E; Virtanen, E; Laine, S; Arvilommi, H. Enhancement of the circulating antibody secreting cell response in human diarrhea by a human Lactobacillus strain. *Pediatr Res*., 1992, 32(2), 141-4. DOI 10.1203/00006450-199208000-00002.

[124] Tozetto-Mendoza, TR; Kanunfre, KA; Vilas-Boas, LS; Sanchez, Espinoza, EP; Paiao, HGO; Rocha, MC; de Paula, AV; de Oliveira, MS; Zampelli, DB; Vieira, JM; Jr. Buss, L; Costa, SF; Sabino, EC; Witkin, SS; Okay, TS; Mendes-Correa, MC. Nucleoprotein-based ELISA for detection of SARS-COV-2 IgG antibodies: Could an old assay be suitable for serodiagnosis of the new coronavirus? *J Virol Methods*., 2021, 290, 114064. DOI 10.1016/j.jviromet.2021.114064.

[125] Friedland, RP; Haribabu, B. The role for the metagenome in the pathogenesis of COVID-19. *EBioMedicine*., 2020, 61, 103019. DOI 10.1016/j.ebiom.2020.103019.

[126] Mostafa, HH; Fissel, JA; Fanelli, B; Bergman, Y; Gniazdowski, V; Dadlani, M; Carroll, KC; Colwell, RR; Simner, PJ. Metagenomic Next-Generation Sequencing of Nasopharyngeal Specimens Collected from Confirmed and Suspect COVID-19 Patients. *mBio*., 2020, 11(6). DOI 10.1128/mBio.01969-20.

[127] Grubaugh, ND; Hodcroft, EB; Fauver, JR; Phelan, AL; Cevik, M. Public health actions to control new SARS-CoV-2 variants. *Cell*., 2021, 184(5), 1127-32. DOI 10.1016/j.cell.2021.01.044.

[128] Zhu, Y; Fu, KW; Grepin, KA; Liang, H; Fung, IC. Limited early warnings and public attention to COVID-19 in China, January-February, 2020: a longitudinal cohort of randomly sampled Weibo users. *Disaster Med Public Health Prep.* 2020;10.1017/dmp.2020.68:1-9. DOI 10.1017/dmp.2020.68.

[129] Caly, L; Druce, J; Roberts, J; Bond, K; Tran, T; Kostecki, R; Yoga, Y; Naughton, W; Taiaroa, G; Seemann, T; Schultz, MB; Howden, BP; Korman, TM; Lewin, SR; Williamson, DA; Catton, MG. Isolation and rapid sharing of the 2019 novel coronavirus (SARS-CoV-2) from the first patient diagnosed with COVID-19 in Australia. *Med J Aust.*, 2020, 10.5694/mja2.50569. DOI 10.5694/mja2.50569.

[130] Pasteur, I. Maladie COVID-19 (Nouveau Coronavirus), 2020, https://www.pasteur.fr/fr/centre-medical/fiches-maladies/maladie-covid-19-nouveau-coronavirus. Available from: https://www.pasteur.fr/fr/centre-medical/fiches-maladies/maladie-covid-19-nouveau-coronavirus.

[131] *Occupational Safety and Health Administration*. 2021 [Available from: https://www.osha.gov/.

[132] Silk, JC. Development of a globally harmonized system for hazard communication. *Int J Hyg Environ Health.,* 2003, 206(4-5), 447-52. DOI 10.1078/1438-4639-00241.

[133] Ta, GC; Jonai, H; Mokhtar, MB; Peterson, PJ. Model for the implementation of the globally harmonized system of classification and labelling of chemicals (GHS): lessons learned from Japan. *J Occup Health.*, 2009, 51(6), 526-30. DOI 10.1539/joh.p9001.

[134] Morita, T; Hayashi, M; Nakajima, M; Tanaka, N; Tweats, DJ; Morikawa, K; Sofuni, T. Practical issues on the application of the GHS classification criteria for germ cell mutagens. *Regul Toxicol Pharmacol.*, 2009, 55(1), 52-68. DOI 10.1016/j.yrtph.2009.06.001.

[135] *CCAC* [Available from: https://www.ccac.ca/en/training/modules/core-stream/occupational-health-and-safety.html.

[136] Lowther, SD; Deng, W; Fang, Z; Booker, D; Whyatt, DJ; Wild, O; Wang, X; Jones, KC. How efficiently can HEPA purifiers remove

priority fine and ultrafine particles from indoor air? *Environ Int.*, 2020, 144, 106001. DOI 10.1016/j.envint.2020.106001.

[137] Zhu, N; Zhang, D; Wang, W; Li, X; Yang, B; Song, J; Zhao, X; Huang, B; Shi, W; Lu, R; Niu, P; Zhan, F; Ma, X; Wang, D; Xu, W; Wu, G; Gao, GF; Tan, W; China Novel Coronavirus, I; Research, T. A Novel Coronavirus from Patients with Pneumonia in China, 2019. *N Engl J Med.*, 2020, 382(8), 727-33. DOI 10.1056/ NEJMoa2001017.

[138] Rachford, BK. The story of quarantine. *J Hist Med Allied Sci.*, 1950, 5(4), 432-43. DOI 10.1093/jhmas/v.autumn.432.

[139] Alfaraj, SH; Al-Tawfiq, JA; Altuwaijri, TA; Alanazi, M; Alzahrani, N; Memish, ZA. Middle East respiratory syndrome coronavirus transmission among health care workers: Implication for infection control. *Am J Infect Control.*, 2018, 46(2), 165-8. DOI 10.1016/ j.ajic.2017.08.010.

[140] Kilwein, JH. Some historical comments on quarantine: Part Two. *J Clin Pharm Ther.,* 1995, 20(5), 249-52. DOI 10.1111/j.1365-2710.1995.tb00658.x.

[141] CDC. U.S. *Quarantine Stations*. 2020; https://www.cdc.gov/ quarantine/quarantine-stations-us.html. Available from: https://www. cdc.gov/quarantine/quarantine-stations-us.html.

[142] Reynolds, C. Quarantine in times of emergency: the scope of s 51(ix) of the Constitution. *J Law Med.,* 2004, 12(2), 166-77. DOI, https://www.ncbi.nlm.nih.gov/pubmed/15575319.

[143] Al-Qahtani, M; AlAli, S; AbdulRahman, A; Salman Alsayyad, A; Otoom, S; Atkin, SL. The prevalence of asymptomatic and symptomatic COVID-19 in a cohort of quarantined subjects. *Int J Infect Dis.,* 2021, 102, 285-8. DOI 10.1016/j.ijid.2020.10.091.

[144] Sanche, S; Lin, YT; Xu, C; Romero-Severson, E; Hengartner, N; Ke, R. High Contagiousness and Rapid Spread of Severe Acute Respiratory Syndrome Coronavirus 2. *Emerg Infect Dis.*, 2020, 26(7). DOI 10.3201/eid2607.200282.

[145] Zarocostas, J. How to fight an infodemic. *Lancet.*, 2020, 395(10225), 676. DOI 10.1016/S0140-6736(20)30461-X.

[146] Sjödin, H; Wilder-Smith, A; Osman, S; Farooq, Z; Rocklöv, J. Only strict quarantine measures can curb the coronavirus disease (COVID-19) outbreak in Italy, 2020. *Euro Surveill.*, 2020, 25(13). DOI https://doi.org/10.2807/1560-7917.ES.2020.25.13.2000280.

[147] DocCheck. *Ich bin es wert, geschützt zu werden* 2020 [Available from: https://www.doccheck.com/de/detail/articles/26464-ich-bin-es-wert-geschuetzt-zu-werden?utm_source=DC-Newsletter& utm_medium=email&utm_campaign=DocCheck-News& utm_content=asset&utm_term=article&sc_src=email_323446&sc_lid=19718799&sc_uid=xrOB0Z7pzf&sc_llid=171015&sc_customer=f68a7adc806cd41162f1a3d19b5d0eb4. [*I am worth protecting*]

[148] Liu, N; Zhang, F; Wei, C; Jia, Y; Shang, Z; Sun, L; Wu, L; Sun, Z; Zhou, Y; Wang, Y; Liu, W. Prevalence and predictors of PTSS during COVID-19 outbreak in China hardest-hit areas: Gender differences matter. *Psychiatry Res.*, 2020, 287, 112921. DOI 10.1016/j.psychres.2020.112921.

[149] Bansal, P; Bingemann, TA; Greenhawt, M; Mosnaim, G; Nanda, A; Oppenheimer, J; Sharma, H; Stukus, D; Shaker, M. Clinician Wellness During the COVID-19 Pandemic: Extraordinary Times and Unusual Challenges for the Allergist/Immunologist. *J Allergy Clin Immunol Pract.*, 2020, 10.1016/j.jaip.2020.04.001. DOI 10.1016/j.jaip.2020.04.001.

[150] Cabas, P; Di Bella, S; Giuffre, M; Rizzo, M; Trombetta, C; Luzzati, R; Antonello, RM; Parenzan, K; Liguori, G. Community pharmacists' exposure to COVID-19. *Res Social Adm Pharm.*, 2021, 17(1), 1882-7. DOI 10.1016/j.sapharm.2020.05.020.

[151] Bong, CL; Brasher, C; Chikumba, E; McDougall, R; Mellin-Olsen, J; Enright, A. The COVID-19 Pandemic: Effects on Low and Middle-Income Countries. *Anesth Analg.*, 2020, 10.1213/ ANE.0000000000004846. DOI 10.1213/ANE.0000000000004846.

[152] Chen, W; Huang, Y. To Protect Healthcare Workers Better, To Save More Lives. *Anesth Analg.,* 2020, 10.1213/ANE.0000000000004834. DOI 10.1213/ANE.0000000000004834.

[153] Feng, S; Shen, C; Xia, N; Song, W; Fan, M; Cowling, BJ. Rational use of face masks in the COVID-19 pandemic. *Lancet Respir Med.*, 2020,10.1016/S2213-2600(20)30134-X. DOI 10.1016/S2213-2600 (20)30134-X.

[154] WHO. *Coronavirus disease (COVID-19) advice for the public. When and how to use masks*. 2020 [April 4, 2020]. Available from: https://www.who.int/emergencies/diseases/novel-coronavirus-2019/advice-for-public/when-and-how-to-use-masks.

[155] WHO. *Advice on the use of masks in the context of COVID-19* (WHO reference number: WHO/2019-nCov/IPC_Masks/2020.4)., 2020 June 5, 2020, (WHO/2019-nCov/IPC_Masks/2020.4).

[156] CDC. *Use of Cloth Face Coverings to Help Slow the Spread of COVID-19.*, 2020 [April 4, 2020]. Available from: https://www.cdc.gov/coronavirus/2019-ncov/prevent-getting-sick/diy-cloth-face-coverings.html.

[157] Ghirardato, P; Maccheroni, F; Marinacci, M. Differentiating ambiguity and ambiguity attitude. *J Econ Theory.*, 2004, 118(2), 133-73. DOI.

[158] Shukman, D. Coronavirus: Expert panel to assess face mask use by public. *BBC News*, 2020. DOI, https://www.bbc.com/news/science-environment-52126735.

[159] Lewis, D. *Is the coronavirus airborne? Experts can't agree* 2020 [updated April 4, 2020April 2, 2020]. Available from: https://www.nature.com/articles/d41586-020-00974-w.

[160] Bourouiba, L. Turbulent Gas Clouds and Respiratory Pathogen Emissions: Potential Implications for Reducing Transmission of COVID-19. *JAMA.*, 2020, 10.1001/jama.2020.4756. DOI 10.1001/jama.2020.4756.

[161] Bin-Reza, F; Lopez Chavarrias, V; Nicoll, A; Chamberland, ME. The use of masks and respirators to prevent transmission of influenza: a systematic review of the scientific evidence. *Influenza Other Respir Viruses.*, 2012, 6(4), 257-67. DOI 10.1111/j.1750-2659.2011.00307.x.

[162] Jefferson, T; Del Mar, C; Dooley, L; Ferroni, E; Al-Ansary, LA; Bawazeer, GA; van Driel, ML; Foxlee, R; Rivetti, A. Physical interventions to interrupt or reduce the spread of respiratory viruses: systematic review. *BMJ.*, 2009, 339, b3675. DOI 10.1136/bmj.b3675.

[163] Jefferson, T; Foxlee, R; Del Mar, C; Dooley, L; Ferroni, E; Hewak, B; Prabhala, A; Nair, S; Rivetti, A. Physical interventions to interrupt or reduce the spread of respiratory viruses: systematic review. *BMJ.*, 2008, 336(7635), 77-80. DOI 10.1136/bmj.39393.510347.BE.

[164] Davies, A; Thompson, KA; Giri, K; Kafatos, G; Walker, J; Bennett, A. Testing the efficacy of homemade masks: would they protect in an influenza pandemic? *Disaster Med Public Health Prep.*, 2013, 7(4), 413-8. DOI 10.1017/dmp.2013.43.

[165] Sim, SW; Moey, KS; Tan, NC. The use of facemasks to prevent respiratory infection: a literature review in the context of the Health Belief Model. *Singapore Med J.*, 2014, 55(3), 160-7. DOI 10.11622/smedj.2014037.

[166] Taylor, M; Raphael, B; Barr, M; Agho, K; Stevens, G; Jorm, L. Public health measures during an anticipated influenza pandemic: Factors influencing willingness to comply. *Risk Manag Healthc Policy.*, 2009, 2, 9-20. DOI 10.2147/RMHP.S4810.

[167] Bae, S; Kim, MC; Kim, JY; Cha, HH; Lim, JS; Jung, J; Kim, MJ; Oh, DK; Lee, MK; Choi, SH; Sung, M; Hong, SB; Chung, JW; Kim, SH. Effectiveness of Surgical and Cotton Masks in Blocking SARS-CoV-2: A Controlled Comparison in 4 Patients. *Ann Intern Med.*, 2020, 10.7326/M20-1342. DOI 10.7326/M20-1342.

[168] Bae, S; Kim, MC; Kim, JY; Cha, HH; Lim, JS; Jung, J; Kim, MJ; Oh, DK; Lee, MK; Choi, SH; Sung, M; Hong, SB; Chung, JW; Kim, SH. Notice of Retraction: Effectiveness of Surgical and Cotton Masks in Blocking SARS-CoV-2. *Ann Intern Med.*, 2020, 10.7326/L20-0745. DOI 10.7326/L20-0745.

[169] Greenhalgh, T; Howard, J. *FastAi* [Internet], 2020. [https://www.fast.ai/2020/04/13/masks-summary/]. Available from: https://www.fast.ai/2020/04/13/masks-summary/.

[170] Carlsten, C; Salvi, S; Wong, GWK; Chung, KF. Personal strategies to minimise effects of air pollution on respiratory health: advice for providers, patients and the public. *Eur Respir J.*, 2020, 10.1183/13993003.02056-2019. DOI 10.1183/13993003.02056-2019.

[171] Tenré, S. *En tissue, chirurgical ou FFP2: à quels masques se fiercontre le Covid-19 ?* Jan 20, 2021. [*In tissue, surgical or FFP2: which masks to trust against Covid-19?*]

[172] Huigang, L; Xiaowei, X; Cui, H; Haixia, M; Zhiming, Y. A brief history of the development of infectious disease prevention, control, and biosafety programs in China. *J Biosaf Biosecur.*, 2020, 2, 23-6. DOI https://doi.org/10.1016/j.jobb.2019.10.002.

[173] Meier, BM. Human Rights in the World Health Organization: Views of the Director-General Candidates. *Health Hum Rights*. 2017, 19(1), 293-8. DOI, https://www.ncbi.nlm.nih.gov/pubmed/28630561.

[174] Ashall, F. Questions around the candidacy of Dr Tedros Adhanom Ghebreyesus for WHO DG. *Lancet.*, 2017, 389(10084), e10. DOI 10.1016/S0140-6736(17)31360-0.

[175] Gostin, LO; Friedman, EA. Reimagining WHO: leadership and action for a new Director-General. *Lancet.*, 2017, 389(10070), 755-9. DOI 10.1016/S0140-6736(17)30203-9.

[176] Cucinotta, D; Vanelli, M. WHO Declares COVID-19 a Pandemic. *Acta Biomed.*. 2020, 91(1), 157-60. DOI 10.23750/abm.v91i1.9397.

[177] Orr, J. First Epistle to the Corinthians. In: Orr J, editor. *The International Standard Bible Encyclopedia*: Wm. B. Eerdmans Publishing; 1995. DOI. https://www.studylight.org/ encyclopedias/ eng/isb/c/corner.html.

[178] Editors. *Herodotus. Encyclopedia Britannica 2019.* DOI. https://www.britannica.com/biography/Herodotus-Greek-historian.

[179] Wilken, R. "John Chrysostom" Profile. In: Ferguson E, editor. *Encyclopedia of Early Christianity*. New York: Garland Publishing, 1997. DOI.

[180] Peters, EN. *The 1917 Pio-Benedictine Code of Canon Law*: Ignatius Press, 2001.

[181] Wesley, J. W*esley's Notes on the Bible: Christian Classics* Ethereal Library, 1987.

[182] Cathcart, L. A milliner's guide to wearing hats in church. *Catholic Herald.* 25 May 2017.

[183] CJW. *Head Coverings - When and Why? Keep Yourselves in God's Love* [Internet]., 2008.

[184] Cross, FL; Livingstone, EA. Matthew, Gospel acc. to St. - The Oxford *Dictionary of the Christian Church.* 3rd ed: Oxford University Press, 2005.

[185] Arnold, DW. *Why I object to Masks, based on Biblical Notions Dean W Arnold* [Internet]., 2020, http://dean-w-arnold.com/articles-blogs/masks. Available from: http://dean-w-arnold.com/articles-blogs/masks.

[186] Best, S. *Wearing Masks & the Bible Highland Heights* [Internet]., 2021 Jan 27, 2021], https://www.hhbc.net/post/wearing-masks-the-bible. Available from: https://www.hhbc.net/post/wearing-masks-the-bible.

[187] Wall, H; Balani, A; Larkin, D. 'Shouting won't help': What psychology can tellus about anti-maskers. *The Independent.*, December 14, 2020.

[188] Crisp, J; Pelletier, D; Duffield, C; Adams, A; Nagy, S. The Delphi method? *Nurs Res.*, 1997, 46(2), 116-8. DOI 10.1097/00006199-199703000-00010.

[189] Sohn, NM. Blame and the couples dynamic. *Focus.*, 1998, 13(5), 5-6. DOI, https://www.ncbi.nlm.nih.gov/pubmed/11365176.

[190] Alia-Klein, N; Gan, G; Gilam, G; Bezek, J; Bruno, A; Denson, TF; Hendler, T; Lowe, L; Mariotti, V; Muscatello, MR; Palumbo, S; Pellegrini, S; Pietrini, P; Rizzo, A; Verona, E. The feeling of anger: From brain networks to linguistic expressions. *Neurosci Biobehav Rev.*, 2020, 108, 480-97. DOI 10.1016/j.neubiorev.2019.12.002.

[191] Qu, W; Dai, M; Zhao, W; Zhang, K; Ge, Y. Expressing Anger Is More Dangerous than Feeling Angry when Driving. *PLoS One.*, 2016, 11(6), e0156948. DOI 10.1371/journal.pone.0156948.

[192] Pasupathi, M; Wainryb, C; Mansfield, CD; Bourne, S. The feeling of the story: Narrating to regulate anger and sadness. *Cogn Emot.*, 2017, 31(3), 444-61. DOI 10.1080/02699931.2015.1127214.

[193] Gino, F; Schweitzer, ME. Blinded by anger or feeling the love: how emotions influence advice taking. *J Appl Psychol.*, 2008, 93(5), 1165-73. DOI 10.1037/0021-9010.93.5.1165.

[194] Désy, J. L'Esprit du Nord.: XYZ, 2015, Nov 13, 2015.

[195] Jakovljevic, M; Jakovljevic, I; Bjedov, S; Mustac, F. Psychiatry for Better World: COVID-19 and Blame Games People Play from Public and Global Metal Health Perspective. *Psychiatr Danub.*, 2020, 32(2), 221-8. DOI 10.24869/psyd.2020.221.

[196] Al-Afnan, MA. COVID-19-The foreign virus: Media bias, ideology and dominance in Chinese and American newspaper articles. *IJALEL* [Internet]., 2020, 9, [56-60 pp.]. Available from: www.ijalel.aiac.org.au.

[197] Trobisch, D. Paul's Letter Collection. Minneapolis: Fortress, 1994.

[198] Nguyen, TT; Criss, S; Dwivedi, P; Huang, D; Keralis, J; Hsu, E; Phan, L; Nguyen, LH; Yardi, I; Glymour, MM; Allen, AM; Chae, DH; Gee, GC; Nguyen, QC. Exploring U.S. Shifts in Anti-Asian Sentiment with the Emergence of COVID-19. *Int J Environ Res Public Health.*, 2020, 17(19). DOI 10.3390/ijerph17197032.

[199] Paradies, Y; Ben, J; Denson, N; Elias, A; Priest, N; Pieterse, A; Gupta, A; Kelaher, M; Gee, G. Racism as a Determinant of Health: A Systematic Review and Meta-Analysis. *PLoS One.*, 2015, 10(9), e0138511. DOI 10.1371/journal.pone.0138511.

[200] Pascoe, EA; Smart Richman, L. Perceived discrimination and health: a meta-analytic review. *Psychol Bull.*, 2009, 135(4), 531-54. DOI 10.1037/a0016059.

[201] Novak, NL; Geronimus, AT; Martinez-Cardoso, AM. Change in birth outcomes among infants born to Latina mothers after a major immigration raid. *Int J Epidemiol.*, 2017, 46(3), 839-49. DOI 10.1093/ije/dyw346.

[202] Nguyen, TT; Adams, N; Huang, D; Glymour, MM; Allen, AM; Nguyen, QC. The Association Between State-Level Racial Attitudes

Assessed From Twitter Data and Adverse Birth Outcomes: Observational Study. *JMIR Public Health Surveill.*, 2020, 6(3), e17103. DOI 10.2196/17103.

[203] Huang, D; Huang, Y; Adams, N; Nguyen, TT; Nguyen, QC. Twitter-Characterized Sentiment Towards Racial/Ethnic Minorities and Cardiovascular Disease (CVD) Outcomes. *J Racial Ethn Health Disparities.*, 2020, 7(5), 888-900. DOI 10.1007/s40615-020-00712-y.

[204] Chae, DH; Clouston, S; Martz, CD; Hatzenbuehler, ML; Cooper, HLF; Turpin, R; Stephens-Davidowitz, S; Kramer, MR. Area racism and birth outcomes among Blacks in the United States. *Soc Sci Med.*, 2018, 199, 49-55. DOI 10.1016/j.socscimed.2017.04.019.

[205] Chae, DH; Clouston, S; Hatzenbuehler, ML; Kramer, MR; Cooper, HL; Wilson, SM; Stephens-Davidowitz, SI; Gold, RS; Link, BG. Association between an Internet-Based Measure of Area Racism and Black Mortality. *PLoS One.*, 2015, 10(4), e0122963. DOI 10.1371/journal.pone.0122963.

[206] Lewis, TT; Cogburn, CD; Williams, DR. Self-reported experiences of discrimination and health: scientific advances, ongoing controversies, and emerging issues. *Annu Rev Clin Psychol.*, 2015, 11, 407-40. DOI 10.1146/annurev-clinpsy-032814-112728.

[207] Lomas, N. *Facebook Users Must Be Allowed to Use Pseudonyms; Says German Privacy Regulator; Real-Name Policy 'Erodes Online Freedoms.*, 2012, Dec 18, 2012, https://techcrunch.com/2012/12/18/facebook-users-must-be-allowed-to-use-pseudonyms-says-german-privacy-regulator-real-name-policy-erodes-online-freedoms/. Available from: https://techcrunch.com/2012/12/18/facebook-users-must-be-allowed-to-use-pseudonyms-says-german-privacy-regulator-real-name-policy-erodes-online-freedoms/.

[208] Kavanaugh, A; Yang, S; Li, LT; Sheetz, S; Fox, E. Microblogging in crisis situations: Mass protests in Iran, Tunisia, Egypt. *CHI* [Internet]., 2011, http://citeseerx.ist.psu.edu/viewdoc/ download?doi=10.1.1.301.9677&rep=rep1&type=pdf. Available from: http://citeseerx.ist.psu.edu/viewdoc/download?doi=10.1.1.301.9677&rep=rep1&type=pdf.

[209] Mustafaraj, E; Metaxas, P; Finn, S; Monroy-Hernandez, A. Hiding in Plain Sight: A Tale of Trust and Mistrust inside a Community of Citizen Reporters. *Proc 6th Int'l AAAI Conf Weblogs and Social Media* (ICWSM 12)., 2012, https://www.aaai.org/ocs/index.php/ICWSM/ICWSM12/paper/viewFile/4677/4990:250-7. DOI.

[210] Suler, J. The online disinhibition effect. *Cyberpsychol Behav.*, 2004, 7(3), 321-6. DOI 10.1089/1094931041291295.

[211] WHO. *Social Stigma Associated with COVID-19.* Available online. 2020. DOI, https://www.who.int/docs/default-source/epi-win/stigma/covid19-stigma-guide.pdf?sfvrsn=48f6ac1_ 2&download=true.

[212] Gee, GC; Ro, MJ; Rimoin, AW. Seven Reasons to Care About Racism and COVID-19 and Seven Things to Do to Stop It. *American Journal of Public Health.*, 2020, 110, 954-5. DOI, https://doi.org/10.2105/AJPH.2020.305712.

[213] LIU PW, LIU, JM. The Dark Side of WeChat. *Monmouth.*, 2020, 32-7.

[214] Davey, G. The China-US blame game: claims-making about the origin of a new virus. *Soc Anthropol.*, 2020, 10.1111/1469-8676.12900. DOI 10.1111/1469-8676.12900.

[215] Verma, R. China's 'mask diplomacy' to change the COVID-19 narrative in Europe. *Asia Eur J.*, 2020, 10.1007/s10308-020-00576-1:1-5. DOI 10.1007/s10308-020-00576-1.

[216] Verma, R. China's diplomacy and changing the COVID-19 narrative. *International Journal: Canada's Journal of Global Policy Analysis.*, 2020, 0, 1-11. DOI 10.1177/0020702020930054.

[217] Lai, G. Scapegoating *Hong Kong's minorities over Covid-19 is dangerous – here's how to avoid it*. Kong Kong Free Press., June 4, 2020.

[218] Erdemir, A; Kowalski, P. *Turkish government scapegoats LGBTI Community for Covid-19 Pandemic.* E-Kathimerini., May 11, 2020.

[219] Rothstein, MA. The Moral Challenge of Ebola. *Am J Public Health.*, 2015, 105(1), 6-8. DOI 10.2105/AJPH.2014.302413.

[220] Bodomo, AB. *Africans in China: A Sociocultural Study and Its Implications on Africa-China Relations*. Amherst, NY: Cambria Press, 2012.

[221] Bogoch, II; Creatore, MI; Cetron, MS; Brownstein, JS; Pesik, N; Miniota, J; Tam, T; Hu, W; Nicolucci, A; Ahmed, S; Yoon, JW; Berry, I; Hay, SI; Anema, A; Tatem, AJ; MacFadden, D; German, M; Khan, K. Assessment of the potential for international dissemination of Ebola virus via commercial air travel during the 2014 west African outbreak. *Lancet.*, 2015, 385(9962), 29-35. DOI 10.1016/S0140-6736(14)61828-6.

[222] WHO. *Ebola virus disease – Democratic Republic of the Congo*. 2020. DOI; https://www.who.int/csr/don/02-january-2020-ebola-drc/en/.

[223] WHO. *Ebola virus disease – Democratic Republic of the Congo*. 2021. DOI, https://www.who.int/csr/don/10-february-2021-ebola-drc/en/#:~:text=On%207%20February%202021%2C%20the,case%20in%20North%20Kivu%20Province.

[224] Ide, W. *Guangzhou hotel serves as China's Ebola quarantine*. . Voice of America [Internet]. 2014 February 1; 2015; https://www.voanews.com/east-asia-pacific/voa-exclusive-guangzhou-hotel-serves-chinas-ebola-quarantine. Available from: https://www.voanews.com/east-asia-pacific/voa-exclusive-guangzhou-hotel-serves-chinas-ebola-quarantine.

[225] Hall, BJ; Chen, W; Latkin, C; Ling, L; Tucker, JD. Africans in south China face social and health barriers. *Lancet.*, 2014, 383(9925), 1291-2. DOI 10.1016/S0140-6736(14)60637-1.

[226] Lin, L; Brown, KB; Yu, F; Yang, J; Wang, J; Schrock, JM; Bodomo, AB; Yang, L; Yang, B; Nehl, EJ; Tucker, JD; Wong, FY. Health Care Experiences and Perceived Barriers to Health Care Access: A Qualitative Study Among African Migrants in Guangzhou, Guangdong Province, China. *J Immigr Minor Health.*, 2015, 17(5), 1509-17. DOI 10.1007/s10903-014-0114-8.

[227] Dirlikov, E; Jiang, Q. *From the dragon's perspective: an initial report on China's response to the unfolding Ebola epidemic*. 2014 February 1, 2015, http://somatosphere.net/2014/10/from-the-dragons

perspective.html. Available from: http://somatosphere.net/ 2014/10/ from-the-dragonsperspective.html.

[228] Lin, L; Hall, BJ; Khoe, LC; Bodomo, AB. Ebola outbreak: from the perspective of African migrants in China. *Am J Public Health.*, 2015, 105(5), e5. DOI 10.2105/AJPH.2015.302649.

[229] HRW. China: Covid-19 Discrimination Against Africans. *Human Rights Watch.*, 2020 May 5, 2020.

[230] Lau, J. *China moves to smooth relations with African students.*, April 20, 2020], https://www.timeshighereducation.com/news/ china-moves-smooth-relations-african-students. Available from: https://www.timeshighereducation.com/news/china-moves-smooth-relations-african-students.

[231] *Racism a 'barrier' for African students in China.*; https:// www.timeshighereducation.com/news/racism-barrier-african-students-china. DOI.

[232] A racist Chinese laundry ad has caused outrage... but Italy did it first. *The Local* (Thelocalit).

[233] Savitsky, S. 'SNL's' Michael Che, NBC accused of 'antisemitic trope' in 'Weekend Update' segment: 'Retract and apologize'. *Fox News.*

[234] Cascio, A; Colomba, C; Di Carlo, P; Serra, N; Lo Re, G; Gambino, A; Lo Casto, A; Guglielmi, G; Veronese, N; Lagalla, R; Sergi, C. Low bone mineral density in HIV-positive young Italians and migrants. *PLoS One.*, 2020, 15(9), e0237984. DOI 10.1371/journal.pone. 0237984.

[235] AAS. Augustinus. *Soliloquiorum Libri Duo, de Inmortalitate Animae, de Quantitate Animae*: Austrian Academy of Sciences Press, 1986, DEc 31, 1986. [*Soliloquiorum Libri Duo, de Inmortalitate Animae, de Quantitate Animae*]

[236] *What is dialogue?*: Clark University; 2021 [Available from: https://www2.clarku.edu/difficultdialogues/learn/index.cfm.

[237] Horowitz, JM; Brown, A; Cox, K. Views on Race in America 2019. *Social & Demographic Trends Project* [Internet]., 2019, 2019-04-09.

[238] Isaac, B. *The Invention of Racism in Classical Antiquity.*: Princeton University Press., 2004.

[239] Wilson, EO. *Sociobiology*. 25 ed: Belknap Press, 2000 03/24/2000. 720 p.

[240] Buck, R. Communicative genes in the evolution of empathy and altruism. *Behav Genet.*, 2011, 41(6), 876-88. DOI 10.1007/s10519-011-9456-3.

[241] Steimer, T. The biology of fear- and anxiety-related behaviors. *Dialogues Clin Neurosci.,* 2002, 4(3), 231-49. DOI; https://www.ncbi.nlm.nih.gov/pubmed/22033741.

[242] Wilson, G. *Feel Better - Create a Scapegoat*. Dr Graham Wilson - 'The Confidant' [Internet]., 2011.

[243] Tacitus, C. *The Annals.* In: Church AJ, Brodribb WJ, editors. XV, http://data.perseus.org/citations/urn:cts:latinLit:phi1351.phi005.perseus-eng1:15.44. New York, NY, U.S.A.: Random House, Inc., 1942.

[244] Campbell, AF; O'Brien, MA. *Sources of the Pentateuch: Texts, Introductions, Annotations*.: Fortress Press, 1993.

[245] Lozano, EB; Laurent, SM. The effect of admitting fault versus shifting blame on expectations for others to do the same. *PLoS One.*, 2019, 14(3), e0213276. DOI 10.1371/journal.pone.0213276.

[246] Shepherd, C; Yang, Y; Seddon, M. WHO investigators deeply sceptical of China's Covid origin theory. *Financial Times.*, 2021, March 2nd, 2021.

[247] Yan, LM; Kang, S; Guan, J; Hu, S. Unusual Features of the SARS-CoV-2 Genome Suggesting Sophisticated Laboratory Modification Rather Than Natural Evolution and Delineation of Its Probable Synthetic Route. *Zenodo* Preprint (https://zenodoorg/record/4028830#YD41YGhKjD7). 2020; https://zenodo.org/record/4028830#.YD41YGhKjD7. DOI.

[248] Zhang, T; Wu, Q; Zhang, Z. Probable Pangolin Origin of SARS-CoV-2 Associated with the COVID-19 Outbreak. *Curr Biol.*, 2020, 30(7), 1346-51 e2. DOI 10.1016/j.cub.2020.03.022.

[249] Science Media Centre [Internet] 2020. [https:// www.sciencemediacentre.org/expert-reaction-to-preprint-entitled-unusual-features-of-the-sars-cov-2-genome-suggesting-sophisticated-laboratory-modification-rather-than-natural-evolution-and-delineation-of-its-

probable-s/]. Available from: https:// www.sciencemediacentre.org/expert-reaction-to-preprint-entitled-unusual-features-of-the-sars-cov-2-genome-suggesting-sophisticated-laboratory-modification-rather-than-natural-evolution-and-delineation-of-its-probable-s/.

[250] Andersen, KG; Rambaut, A; Lipkin, WI; Holmes, EC; Garry, RF. The proximal origin of SARS-CoV-2. *Nat Med.*, 2020, 26(4), 450-2. DOI 10.1038/s41591-020-0820-9.

[251] Seyran, M; Pizzol, D; Adadi, P; El-Aziz, TMA; Hassan, SS; Soares, A; Kandimalla, R; Lundstrom, K; Tambuwala, M; Aljabali, AAA; Lal, A; Azad, GK; Choudhury, PP; Uversky, VN; Sherchan, SP; Uhal, BD; Rezaei, N; Brufsky, AM. Questions concerning the proximal origin of SARS-CoV-2. *J Med Virol.*, 2021, 93(3), 1204-6. DOI 10.1002/jmv.26478.

[252] Wakefield, AJ; Murch, SH; Anthony, A; Linnell, J; Casson, DM; Malik, M; Berelowitz, M; Dhillon, AP; Thomson, MA; Harvey, P; Valentine, A; Davies, SE; Walker-Smith, JA. Ileal-lymphoid-nodular hyperplasia, non-specific colitis, and pervasive developmental disorder in children. *Lancet.*, 1998, 351(9103), 637-41. DOI 10.1016/s0140-6736(97)11096-0.

[253] Leung, AK; Hon, KL; Leong, KF; Sergi, CM. Measles: a disease often forgotten but not gone. *Hong Kong Med J.*, 2018, 24(5), 512-20. DOI 10.12809/hkmj187470.

[254] Taylor, LE; Swerdfeger, AL; Eslick, GD. Vaccines are not associated with autism: an evidence-based meta-analysis of case-control and cohort studies. *Vaccine.*, 2014, 32(29), 3623-9. DOI 10.1016/j.vaccine.2014.04.085,

[255] Bavel, JJV; Baicker, K; Boggio, PS; Capraro, V; Cichocka, A; Cikara, M; Crockett, MJ; Crum, AJ; Douglas, KM; Druckman, JN; Drury, J; Dube, O; Ellemers, N; Finkel, EJ; Fowler, JH; Gelfand, M; Han, S; Haslam, SA; Jetten, J; Kitayama, S; Mobbs, D; Napper, LE; Packer, DJ; Pennycook, G; Peters, E; Petty, RE; Rand, DG; Reicher, SD; Schnall, S; Shariff, A; Skitka, LJ; Smith, SS; Sunstein, CR; Tabri, N; Tucker, JA; Linden, SV; Lange, PV; Weeden, KA; Wohl MJA; Zaki, J; Zion, SR; Willer, R. Using social and behavioural science to support

COVID-19 pandemic response. *Nat Hum Behav.*, 2020, 4(5), 460-71. DOI 10.1038/s41562-020-0884-z.

[256] Zhou, P; Huang, Z; Xiao, Y; Huang, X; Fan, XG. Protecting Chinese Healthcare Workers While Combating the 2019 Novel Coronavirus. *Infect Control Hosp Epidemiol.*, 2020, 10.1017/ice.2020.60:1-4. DOI 10.1017/ice.2020.60.

[257] Goodman, JC. The Dangers In Nationalizing Health Care. *Forbes.*, 2020, Feb 12, 2020.

[258] Galton, F. *Inquiries into Human Faculty and its Development*. London, UK: Macmillan, 1883.

[259] Holmes, OW; Court, US. *Buck v. Bell. US Reports* [Internet]., 1926, 274(200). Available from: https://www.loc.gov/item/usrep274200/.

[260] U.S. District Court WDVLD. Poe v. Lynchburg Training School and Hospital. *Fed Suppl.*, 1981, 518, 789-94. DOI, https://www.ncbi.nlm.nih.gov/pubmed/11648518.

[261] Benedek, TG. The 'Tuskegee Study' of syphilis: analysis of moral versus methodologic aspects. *J Chronic Dis.*, 1978, 31(1), 35-50. DOI 10.1016/0021-9681(78)90079-6.

[262] Brandon, DT; Isaac, LA; LaVeist, TA. The legacy of Tuskegee and trust in medical care: is Tuskegee responsible for race differences in mistrust of medical care? *J Natl Med Assoc.*, 2005, 97(7), 951-6. DOI, https://www.ncbi.nlm.nih.gov/pubmed/16080664.

[263] Brandt, AM. Racism and research: the case of the Tuskegee Syphilis Study. *Hastings Cent Rep.*, 1978, 8(6), 21-9. DOI; https://www.ncbi.nlm.nih.gov/pubmed/721302.

[264] Corbie-Smith, G. The continuing legacy of the Tuskegee Syphilis Study: considerations for clinical investigation. *Am J Med Sci.*, 1999, 317(1), 5-8. DOI 10.1097/00000441-199901000-00002.

[265] Freimuth, VS; Quinn, SC; Thomas, SB; Cole, G; Zook, E; Duncan, T. African Americans' views on research and the Tuskegee Syphilis Study. *Soc Sci Med.*, 2001, 52(5), 797-808. DOI 10.1016/s0277-9536(00)00178-7.

[266] Katz, RV; Kegeles, SS; Green, BL; Kressin, NR; James, SA; Claudio, C. The Tuskegee Legacy Project: history, preliminary scientific

findings, and unanticipated societal benefits. *Dent Clin North Am.*, 2003, 47(1), 1-19. DOI 10.1016/s0011-8532(02)00049-6.

[267] Schmidt, TA. The legacy of the Tuskegee syphilis experiments for emergency exception from informed consent. *Ann Emerg Med.*, 2003, 41(1), 79-81. DOI 10.1067/mem.2003.17.

[268] Sencer, DJ; Millar, JD. Reflections on the 1976 swine flu vaccination program. *Emerg Infect Dis.*, 2006, 12(1), 29-33. DOI 10.3201/eid1201.051007.

[269] Harris, K. Legislation to expand access to medically assisted death clears House, moves to Senate. *CBC News.*, Dec 10, 2020.

[270] Williams, OD. COVID-19 and Private Health: Market and Governance Failure. *Development* (Rome)., 2020, 10.1057/s41301-020-00273-x:1-10. DOI 10.1057/s41301-020-00273-x.

[271] Pottie, K; Hui, C; Rahman, P; Ingleby, D; Akl, EA; Russell, G; Ling, L; Wickramage, K; Mosca, D; Brindis, CD. Building Responsive Health Systems to Help Communities Affected by Migration: An International Delphi Consensus. *Int J Environ Res Public Health.*, 2017, 14(2). DOI 10.3390/ijerph14020144.

[272] Wedlake, M. COVID-19 and mental health: Feeling anguish is normal and is not a disorder. *The Conversation* [Internet]. 2021 Mar 9; 2021; https://theconversation.com/covid-19-and-mental-health-feeling-anguish-is-normal-and-is-not-a-disorder-153784. Available from: https://theconversation.com/covid-19-and-mental-health-feeling-anguish-is-normal-and-is-not-a-disorder-153784.

[273] *CDC.* [Available from: https://www.cdc.gov/media/releases/2020/p1218-overdose-deaths-covid-19.html.

[274] Volpe, DA; McMahon Tobin, GA; Mellon, RD; Katki, AG; Parker, RJ; Colatsky, T; Kropp, TJ; Verbois, SL. Uniform assessment and ranking of opioid mu receptor binding constants for selected opioid drugs. *Regul Toxicol Pharmacol.*, 2011, 59(3), 385-90. DOI 10.1016/j.yrtph.2010.12.007

[275] Sato, S; Suzuki, S; Lee, XP; Sato, K. Studies on 1-(2-phenethyl)-4-(N-propionylanilino)piperidine (fentanyl) and related compounds VII. Quantification of alpha-methylfentanyl metabolites excreted in rat

urine. *Forensic Sci Int.*, 2010, 195(1-3), 68-72. DOI 10.1016/j.forsciint.2009.11.014.

[276] Nelson, L; Schwaner, R. Transdermal fentanyl: pharmacology and toxicology. *J Med Toxicol.*, 2009, 5(4), 230-41. DOI 10.1007/BF03178274.

[277] Rose, ME. Are Prescription Opioids Driving the Opioid Crisis? Assumptions vs Facts. *Pain Med.*, 2018, 19(4), 793-807. DOI 10.1093/pm/pnx048.

[278] Stoecker, WV; Bosworth, KT; Rottnek, F. Missouri's Fentanyl Problem: The China Connection. *Mo Med.,* 2020, 117(4), 362-9. DOI, https://www.ncbi.nlm.nih.gov/pubmed/32848274.

[279] Smith, MJ; Cobia, DJ; Reilly, JL; Gilman, JM; Roberts, AG; Alpert, KI; Wang, L; Breiter, HC; Csernansky, JG. Cannabis-related episodic memory deficits and hippocampal morphological differences in healthy individuals and schizophrenia subjects. *Hippocampus.*, 2015, 25(9), 1042-51. DOI 10.1002/hipo.22427.

[280] Badowski, ME. A review of oral cannabinoids and medical marijuana for the treatment of chemotherapy-induced nausea and vomiting: a focus on pharmacokinetic variability and pharmacodynamics. *Cancer Chemother Pharmacol.*, 2017, 80(3), 441-9. DOI 10.1007/s00280-017-3387-5.

[281] Hill, KP. Medical Marijuana for Treatment of Chronic Pain and Other Medical and Psychiatric Problems: A Clinical Review. *JAMA.*, 2015, 313(24), 2474-83. DOI 10.1001/jama.2015.6199.

[282] Choo, EK; Feldstein Ewing, SW; Lovejoy, TI. Opioids Out, Cannabis In: Negotiating the Unknowns in Patient Care for Chronic Pain. *JAMA.*, 2016, 316(17), 1763-4. DOI 10.1001/ jama.2016.13677.

[283] Corroon, J; Sexton, M; Bradley, R. Indications and administration practices amongst medical cannabis healthcare providers: a cross-sectional survey. *BMC Fam Pract.*, 2019, 20(1), 174. DOI 10.1186/s12875-019-1059-8.

[284] Morales, P; Reggio, PH; Jagerovic, N. An Overview on Medicinal Chemistry of Synthetic and Natural Derivatives of Cannabidiol. *Front Pharmacol.*, 2017, 8, 422. DOI 10.3389/fphar.2017.00422.

[285] Dobs, YE; Ali, MM. The epigenetic modulation of alcohol/ethanol and cannabis exposure/co-exposure during different stages. *Open Biol.*, 2019, 9(1),180115. DOI 10.1098/rsob.180115.

[286] Ghasemiesfe, M; Barrow, B; Leonard, S; Keyhani, S; Korenstein, D. Association Between Marijuana Use and Risk of Cancer: A Systematic Review and Meta-analysis. *JAMA Netw Open.*, 2019, 2(11), e1916318. DOI 10.1001/jamanetworkopen.2019.16318.

[287] Deshpande, A; Mailis-Gagnon, A; Zoheiry, N; Lakha, SF. Efficacy and adverse effects of medical marijuana for chronic noncancer pain: Systematic review of randomized controlled trials. *Can Fam Physician.*, 2015, 61(8), e372-81. DOI; https://www.ncbi.nlm.nih.gov/pubmed/26505059.

[288] Hill, KP; Palastro, MD; Johnson, B; Ditre, JW. Cannabis and Pain: A Clinical Review. *Cannabis Cannabinoid Res.*, 2017, 2(1), 96-104. DOI 10.1089/can.2017.0017.

[289] Meier, MH; Caspi, A; Cerda, M; Hancox, RJ; Harrington, H; Houts, R; Poulton, R; Ramrakha, S; Thomson, WM; Moffitt, TE. Associations Between Cannabis Use and Physical Health Problems in Early Midlife: A Longitudinal Comparison of Persistent Cannabis vs Tobacco Users. *JAMA Psychiatry.*, 2016, 73(7), 731-40. DOI 10.1001/jamapsychiatry.2016.0637.

[290] Cerrelli, G; Invernizzi, M. *La famiglia in italia dal divorzio al gender*: Sugarco Edizioni, 2017. [*The family in Italy from divorce to gender*]

[291] Andreazza M. Giuseppe Toniolo. *Un laico Cristiano, un docente, un testimone.* Pisa: ETS Press, 1988. [*A lay Christian, a teacher, a witness*.]

[292] D'Avila, T. *Camino de Perfección* [*The Way of Perfection*], 1577.

[293] McCormick, P. *Sin As Addiction*. New York: Paulist Press, 1989.

[294] Gamble, HY. *Books and Readers in the Early Church: A History of Early Christian Texts.*: Yale University Press, 1995.

[295] Morris, RB. *Seven Who Shaped Our Destiny: The Founding Fathers as Revolutionaries.* 1st ed. New York: Harper & Row, 1973.

[296] Mein, SA. COVID-19 and Health Disparities: the Reality of "the Great Equalizer". *J Gen Intern Med.*, 2020, 35(8), 2439-40. DOI 10.1007/s11606-020-05880-5.

[297] Von Bingen, H. *Worte lebendigen Lichts Freiburg im Breisgau*, Germany: Verlag Herder GmbH, 2012. [*Words of Living Light Freiburg im Breisgau*]

[298] Desmond, A; Offit, PA. On the Shoulders of Giants - From Jenner's Cowpox to mRNA Covid Vaccines. *N Engl J Med.*, 2021, 384(12), 1081-3. DOI 10.1056/NEJMp2034334.

[299] Dan, JM; Mateus, J; Kato, Y; Hastie, KM; Yu, ED; Faliti, CE; Grifoni, A; Ramirez, SI; Haupt, S; Frazier, A; Nakao, C; Rayaprolu, V; Rawlings, SA; Peters, B; Krammer, F; Simon, V; Saphire, EO; Smith, DM; Weiskopf, D; Sette, A; Crotty, S. Immunological memory to SARS-CoV-2 assessed for up to 8 months after infection. *Science.*, 2021, 371(6529). DOI 10.1126/science.abf4063.

[300] Widge, AT; Rouphael, NG; Jackson, LA; Anderson, EJ; Roberts, PC; Makhene, M; Chappell, JD; Denison, MR; Stevens, LJ; Pruijssers, AJ; McDermott, AB; Flach, B; Lin, BC; Doria-Rose, NA; O'Dell, S; Schmidt, SD; Neuzil, KM; Bennett, H; Leav, B; Makowski, M; Albert, J; Cross, K; Edara, VV; Floyd, K; Suthar, MS; Buchanan, W; Luke, CJ; Ledgerwood, JE; Mascola, JR; Graham, BS; Beigel, JH. m RNASG. Durability of Responses after SARS-CoV-2 mRNA-1273 Vaccination. *N Engl J Med.*, 2021, 384(1), 80-2. DOI 10.1056/NEJMc2032195.

[301] Sergi, CM; Leung, A. Vaccination: a question of social responsibility. *J Prev Med Hyg.*, 2021, https://doi.org/ 10.15167/2421-4248/jpmh2021.62.1.1736(62):E46-E7. DOI.

[302] Abbasi, J. COVID-19 and mRNA Vaccines-First Large Test for a New Approach. *JAMA.*, 2020, 324(12), 1125-7. DOI 10.1001/jama.2020.16866.

[303] Parry, J. Covid-19: Hong Kong scientists report first confirmed case of reinfection. *BMJ.*, 2020, 370:m3340. DOI 10.1136/bmj.m3340.

[304] Jensen, J. A Review of Public–Private Partnership Activities in Health System Strengthening. In: Jensen J, editor. *The Role of Public-Private*

Partnerships in Health Systems Strengthening: Workshop Summary. The National Academies Collection: Reports funded by National Institutes of Health, 10.17226/21861. Washington (DC): National Academies Press, 2016.

[305] Girard, R. L'humiliante absence d'un vaccin français. *Le Figaro.,* 2021 February 16, 2021. [The humiliating absence of a French vaccine.]

[306] Schraer, R. Covid-19: Vaccine as good in 'real world' as in trial in Israel. *BBC News.*, 2021 February 15, 2021.

[307] Bridle, BW. 5 factors that could dictate the success or failure of the COVID-19 vaccine rollout. *The Conversation.*, 2021 2/11/2021.

[308] Leung, AKC; Leong, KF; Sergi, CM. Morbilliform rash and conjunctival injection in a febrile child. *Paediatr Child Health.*, 2020, 25(8), 481-2. DOI 10.1093/pch/pxz100.

[309] Leung, AKC; Hon, KL; Leong, KF. Rubella (German measles) revisited. *Hong Kong Med J.*, 2019, 25(2), 134-41. DOI 10.12809/ hkmj187785.

[310] Leung, AKC; Sergi, CM; Lam, JM; Leong, KF. Gianotti-Crosti syndrome (papular acrodermatitis of childhood) in the era of a viral recrudescence and vaccine opposition. *World J Pediatr.*, 2019, 10.1007/s12519-019-00269-9. DOI 10.1007/s12519-019-00269-9.

[311] Amanat, F; Krammer, F. SARS-CoV-2 Vaccines: Status Report. *Immunity.*, 2020, 10.1016/j.immuni.2020.03.007. DOI 10.1016/j. immuni.2020.03.007.

[312] Patsali, ME; Mousa, DV; Papadopoulou, EVK; Papadopoulou, KKK; Kaparounaki, CK; Diakogiannis, I; Fountoulakis, KN. University students' changes in mental health status and determinants of behavior during the COVID-19 lockdown in Greece. *Psychiatry Res.,* 2020, 292, 113298. DOI 10.1016/ j.psychres.2020.113298.

[313] Friedman, RA. Why Humans Are Vulnerable to Conspiracy Theories. *Psychiatr Serv.*, 2020, 10.1176/ appi.ps.202000348 :appips2020 00348. DOI 10.1176/ appi.ps.202000348.

[314] Hiller, KM; Sullivan, D. Influenza vaccination in the emergency department: are our patients at risk? *J Emerg Med.*, 2009, 37(4), 439-43. DOI 10.1016/j.jemermed.2008.08.023.

[315] WHO. *Top ten threats to global health in 2019.*: World Health Organization; 2019 [Available from: https://www.who.int/emergencies/ten-threats-to-global-health-in-2019.

[316] UN. *International Covenant on Economic, Social and Cultural Rights.*: United Nations Human Rights, Office of the High Commissioner; 1966 [Available from: https://www.ohchr.org/en/professionalinterest/pages/cescr.aspx.

[317] Zialcita, P. Facebook Pays $643,000 Fine For Role In Cambridge Analytica Scandal. *NPR.*, October 30, 2019.

[318] Kitchener, KS. Intuition, critical evaluation and ethical principles: The foundation for ethical decisions in counseling psychology. *The Counseling Psychologist.*, 1984, 12(3-4), 43-55. DOI.

[319] Biden has assembled a stellar science team - now they must pull together. *Nature.*, 2021, 590(7844), 7-8. DOI 10.1038/d41586-021-00184-y.

[320] How Joe Biden plans to heal American healthcare. *BMJ.*, 2021, 372, n176. DOI 10.1136/bmj.n176

[321] Berenson, R. Medicare's Stewardship Role to Improve Care Delivery: Opportunities for the Biden Administration. *J Health Polit Policy Law.*, 2021, 10.1215/03616878-8970838. DOI 10.1215/03616878-8970838.

[322] Carter, JM; Goldman, GT; Rosenberg, AA; Reed, G; Desikan, A; MacKinney, T. Strengthen scientific integrity under the Biden administration. *Science.*, 2021, 371(6530), 668-71. DOI 10.1126/science.abg0533.

[323] Dusetzina, SB. Cancer Care Under the Biden Administration. *JAMA.*, 2021, 325(6), 527-8. DOI 10.1001/jama.2020.25424.

[324] Editorial. Biden time. *Nat Phys.*, 2021, 17, 147. DOI; https://doi.org/10.1038/s41567-021-01183-6.

[325] Jaffe, S. Biden unwinds Trump health-care policies. *Lancet.*, 2021, 397(10272), 362-3. DOI 10.1016/S0140-6736(21)00182-3.

[326] Mervis, J. Biden breaks new ground with science team picks. *Science.*, 2021, 371(6528), 452-3. DOI 10.1126/science.371.6528.452

[327] Oberlander, J. Introduction: Health Policy and the Biden Administration. *J Health Polit Policy Law.*, 2021, 10.1215/03616878-8970725. DOI 10.1215/03616878-8970725.

[328] The Lancet Respiratory M. The Biden administration: changing the tide for health? *Lancet Respir Med.*, 2021, 10.1016/S2213-2600(21)00078-3. DOI 10.1016/S2213-2600(21)00078-3.

[329] Weitzman, C; Augustyn, M; Froehlich, T; Mehlenbeck, R; Mendelsohn, AL; Nielsen, BA; Soares, N; Voigt, RG; Walton, J; Zlomke, K; Fogler, J; Keder, RD; Ratliff-Schaub, K; Wallis, KE. Recommendations for the Biden-Harris Administration. A Statement of Priorities from the Society for Developmental and Behavioral Pediatrics. *J Dev Behav Pediatr.*. 2021, 42(2), 152-3. DOI 10.1097/DBP.0000000000000917.

[330] Australia news code: What's this row with Facebook and Google all about? *BBC News.*, 2021, Feb 18, 2021.

[331] Constantinidou, S. Helen and Pandora: A Comparative Study with Emphasis on the *Eidolon* theme as a concept of *Eris.*, [165-241 pp.].

[332] Polkinghorne, D. *Practice and the Human Sciences: The Case for a Judgment-Based Practice of Care.*: SUNY Press, 2004.

[333] John Dryden, J. Hugh Clough A. *Plutarch's Lives.*, 1859.

[334] Möller, M. *Talis oratio – qualis vita. Zu Theorie und Praxis mimetischer Verfahren in der griechisch-römischen Literaturkritik.* Heidelberg; Germany: Universitatsverlag Winter; 2004. [*Talis oratio - qualis vita. On the theory and practice of mimetic procedures in Greco-Roman literary criticism.*]

[335] Abbott, E. Charles Booth, 1840-1916. *Journal of Political Economy.*, 1917, 25(2), 195-200. DOI 10.1086/252946.

[336] Unknown. *Revolutionary Ideals are Higher than Heaven-Studying Comrade Xi Jinping's Important Elaboration concerning Strengthening Ideals and Convictions.* China Copyright and Media., 2013. DOI.

[337] Hobbes, T. *Leviathan or The Matter, Forme and Power of a Commonwealth Ecclesiasticall and Civil.* England, 1651.

[338] Plautus, TM. *Asinaria. Madison, Wisconsin*: University of Wisconsin Press, 2006, 2006.

[339] Harper, J. *Beijing now has more billionaires than any city.*, 2021, https://www.bbc.com/news/business-56671638#:~:text=Beijing's%20richest%20resident%20was%20Zhang;a%20fortune%20worth%20%2459bn. Available from: https:// www.bbc.com/news/business-56671638#:~:text=Beijing's%20richest%20resident%20was%20Zhang;a%20fortune%20worth%20%2459bn.

[340] Marwaha, S. Todor. *Canadian Medical Association Journal.*, 2021, 193(7), E259-E. DOI 10.1503/cmaj.210167.

[341] BMJVS. *Solidaritätszuschlaggesetz 1995 (§4 SolzG).* Bundesminist. Justiz u. f. Verbraucherschutz; 1995. DOI; https://www.gesetze-im-internet.de/solzg_1995/__4.html. [*Solidarity Surcharge Act 1995 (§4 SolzG).*]

[342] Hawes, J. The shortest history of Germany.: *The Experiment*, 2019, March 19; 2019.

[343] Cruickshank, J. Albert Camus. *Encyclopedia Britannica 2021.* DOI; https://www.britannica.com/biography/Albert-Camus.

[344] Shuster, S. Camus's L'etranger and the first description of a man with Asperger's syndrome. *Psychol Res Behav Manag.*, 2018, 11, 117-21. DOI 10.2147/PRBM.S157669.

[345] Slochower, H. Camus' The Stranger: the silent society and the ecstasy of rage. *Am Imago.*, 1969, 26(3), 291-4. DOI; https://www.ncbi.nlm.nih.gov/pubmed/4908191.

[346] Stamm, JL. Camus' Stranger: his act of violence. *Am Imago.*, 1969, 26(3), 281-90. DOI; https://www.ncbi.nlm.nih.gov/pubmed/4908190.

[347] Camus, A. L'Étranger: *Gallimard*, 1942, 159 p.

[348] Balboa, R. Rocky Balboa. In: Stallone S, editor. *United States of America*, 2006. DOI,

[349] Nodé-Langlois, F. Chunyan Li: Finalement, la France est plus socialiste que la Chine!. *Le Figaro*. March 1st, 2021. [Finally, France is more socialist than China!]

[350] Socci, A. *Lo Straniero* [Internet]. Socci A, editor2021. [cited 2021 April 14, 2021]. Available from: https://www.antoniosocci.com/papa-bergoglio-discute-di-proprieta-privata-altrui-e-comunismo-ma-ce-un-problema/. [*The stranger*]

[351] Carlson, T. Mainstream media disinformation more powerful and destructive than QAnon. *Fox News.*, 2021 February 23; 2021.

[352] Carlson, B. *Ben Carson's appeal to the American people: Stop listening to media foolishness.* 2021. DOI.

[353] Bruno G. Spaccio de la Bestia Trionfante1584.

[354] Britannica. Afonso I. *Encyclopedia Britannica.* London, United Kingdom: *Encyclopedia Britannica*, Inc.; 2021. DOI, https://www.britannica.com/biography/Afonso-I-king-of-Kongo-kingdom.

[355] FSSP. Afonso I: the Constantine of the Congo. *The Missive* [Internet]. 2020 Feb 13, 2021, https://fssp.com/afonso-i-the-constantine-of-the-congo/. Available from: https://fssp.com/afonso-i-the-constantine-of-the-congo/.

[356] Frankl, VE. *Man's Search for Meaning. An Introduction to Logotherapy.* Boston, MA: Beacon, 2006.

[357] Fein, EB. New York Times, 11-20-1991. *The New York Times.*, 1991 20 November 1991.

[358] Wilner, J. *You have a Calling* [Internet] 2021. [cited 2021]. Available from: https://youhaveacalling.com/personal-success/10-tips-to-find-meaning-and-hope-during-times-of-despair.

[359] Chalfant, M. Biden scolds Republicans for not wearing masks during Capitol attack. *The Hill.*, 2021, January 15, 2021.

[360] Argandona, A. *The Logic of Gift in Business*: IEDE Business School University of Navarra, 2011.

[361] Wagner, WJ. In Gratitude for What We Are Given: A Common Morality for the Global Age. *J Law; Phil & Culture.*, 2009, 11(1), 7-53. DOI;

[362] Ratzinger, J. The Morality of Exile: Biblical Aspects of the Theme of Faith and Politics. In: Scott D; editor. *Liturgy and Empire: Faith in Exile and Political Theology: St. Paul Center for Biblical Theology*, 2009, p. 286.

Author's Contact Information

Consolato M. Sergi
Full Professor of Pathology and Pediatrics,
University of Alberta, Canada
Children's Hospital of Eastern Ontario,
University of Ottawa, ON, Canada
http://orcid.org/0000-0002-2779-7879
sergi@ualberta.ca

INDEX

R

S

T

V

W